Ayurvedic Massage

Other books by Harish Johari

Attunements for Dawn and Dusk (audiocassettes)

The Birth of the Ganga

Breath, Mind, and Consciousness

Chakras

Chants to the Sun and Moon (audiocassette)

Dhanwantari

The Healing Cuisine

The Healing Power of Gemstones

Leela

The Monkeys and the Mango Tree

Numerología

Numerology

The Planet Meditation Kit

Respiración, mente y conciencia

Sounds of Tantra (audiocassettes)

Sounds of the Chakras (audiocassette)

Tools for Tantra

Ayurvedic Massage

Traditional Indian Techniques for Balancing Body and Mind

HARISH JOHARI

Illustrations by
PIETER WELTEVREDE

Healing Arts Press
Rochester, Vermont

Healing Arts Press
One Park Street
Rochester, Vermont 05767
www.InnerTraditions.com

Healing Arts Press is a division of Inner Traditions International

*Note to the reader: This book is intended as an informational guide. The remedies,
approaches, and techniques described herein are meant to supplement, and not to be a
substitute for, professional medical care or treatment. They should not be used to treat a
serious ailment without prior consultation with a qualified health care professional.*

Library of Congress Cataloging-in-Publication Data

Johari, Harish, 1934–
Ayurvedic massage: traditional Indian techniques for balancing
body and mind / Harish Johari ; illustrations by Pieter Weltevrede.
p. cm.
Includes index.
ISBN 0-89281-489-6
1. Massage therapy. 2. Medicine, Ayurvedic. I. Title.
RM721. J64 1996
615.8'22—dc20   96-16436
                                                      CIP

Printed and bound in the United States

10 9 8 7

Text design and layout by Kathryn Miles Schenkman
This book was typeset in Minion with Shelley Andante Script and Weiss
as the display fonts

Contents

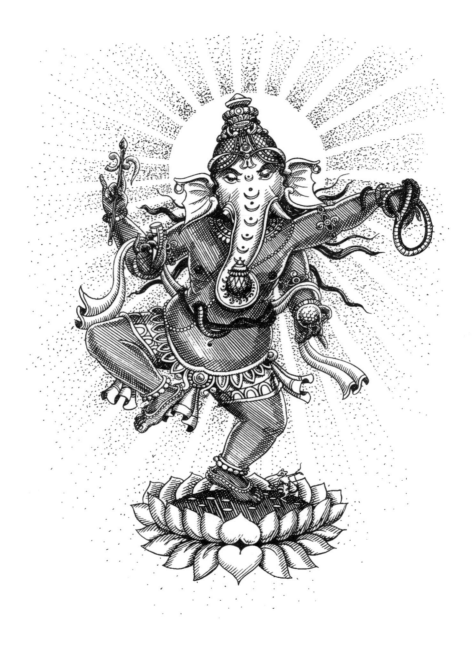

𝒫reface

My training in Ayurveda started at an early age. As a child of eight or ten, I would assist my mother in making powdered herbal remedies, healing poultices, face masks, and herbal teas. Later on I would assist my grandfather and granduncle in making eye remedies, oxides and pastes from gemstones, and rejuvenating tonics *(rasayanas)*.

Between the years 1955 and 1968 I was in the constant company of an Ayurvedic practitioner, a *vaidya,* by the name of Rameshwar Prasad Pande. During this period, I learned about the healing energy of foods, herbs, plants, and gemstones; the *doshas* or body humors; the role of astrology in understanding illness (both physical and mental); and how to detect disease by examining various parts of the body. My interest in Tantric yoga and alchemy brought me to meet many vaidyas, and each of them taught me something valuable about life.

At the age of thirteen I became a regular practitioner of wrestling. At the martial arts school, or *akhara,* in Jaunpur I met many vaidyas who practiced wrestling for their own physical and mental well-being. Wrestlers in India could be called the artists of bodywork—they work with prana, pranic energy, breath control,* and various exercises to build strength, stamina, and vigor. Massage was an integral part of wrestling.

In ancient times Ayurvedic clinics did not regularly offer massage, as everybody gave and received massage. Whenever patients needed a particular treatment they were referred by vaidyas to massage specialists. These technicians used special oils and rubbed the afflicted areas as instructed by the Ayurvedic doctor. Often these massage practitioners were wrestlers. Today in India massage practitioners with this training roam public places in great number and give head and body massages for a few rupees. Although they may have no knowledge of Ayurveda, they do know how to work with muscles, joints, and

---

* This is not the same as the pranayama techniques taught in yoga.

bones. One of my trainers was the famous wrestler Siddique Khan, from Nawab of Rampur. He was a perfected master of massage who could heal and strengthen any body part, tissue, or muscle.

Some of these wrestlers/massage practitioners were also Ayurvedic doctors and/or *hakims*. (A hakim is a doctor who has studied the Unani [Greek] system of medicine.) Over time they developed a special system of their own that contained the knowledge of the Ayurvedic or Unani system of medicine. The massage methods described in this book are based on the techniques of these doctor/wrestlers. I call it traditional Indian massage based on Ayurvedic principles, such as the doshas and *marmas* (pressure points). Over the years I have trained with two main groups of teachers, one Hindu and the other Muslim. From the Hindu teachers I learned about marmas and doshas; from the Muslims I learned about pressure points called *muqame makhsoos*. Much of the time the marmas and the muqame makhsoos are the same, but there are occasional important and helpful differences. Some of the pressure points on the feet correspond to those used in the West by reflexologists.

The massage presented in this book is primarily preventive and is to be practiced on a regular basis for this purpose. Except for dealing with some minor ailments, this massage method is not meant to be therapeutic. It is not, for example, the same as the massage given before *panchakarma* (purification) treatments. Many therapeutic Ayurvedic methods use oils and techniques specific to a particular disease condition. These methods should be practiced only under the supervision of an Ayurvedic doctor or vaidya, and they are not covered in this book.

∼❦∼

I thank my guides, teachers, and students who helped me create this book. I hope it will be of some practical use to those interested in improving their mental and physical well-being.

Introduction

*M*an's strongest desire is to live a healthy, happy, and inspired life. Of these three, health is primary because without it one cannot feel happy or inspired. One of the keys to good health is having a body that circulates nutrients properly and expels toxins efficiently. Food provides us with the proper nutrients, exercise and massage supply the proper circulation, and massage helps our bodies grow and renew. Massage also provides relaxation. By enhancing the circulation of nutrient material and helping the organism expel toxins, massage plays an important role in cleansing and maintaining the health of the body. This cleansing role is what makes massage a most beneficial practice for achieving inspiration and joy. It excites the body's internal resources, stimulating it to process protein, convert various forms of sugar into glucose, and generate various chemical enzymes. If adopted as a daily practice, massage can help rejuvenate the body.

In India massages are given from the time of birth. Babies are regularly massaged with oil, even when they cry. A mother knows that massage will enhance circulation in her infant, who, although continually moving, is unable to perform exercises of any kind. Children are massaged regularly each day until the age of three. Then the routine changes and massage is given once or twice a week, until the child reaches six years of age. At this point, the child is old enough to give and exchange massages with others.

Eighty percent of the population in India live in villages where this tradition is still alive. In rural areas, weekly massage is a family scene—everyone does it. With the hectic pace of life in large towns and cities, it is becoming increasingly difficult to maintain this tradition. However, even in big cities like Delhi, Bombay, and Calcutta, a massage man can often be seen with his mat and a rack of small oil bottles practicing his trade in the park or on the beach. People in India enjoy being massaged; they know that, like a best friend, it brings joy and relaxation.

In India, temple sculptures, calendars, and illustrated spiritual books often depict Vishnu, the lord of preservation, reclining on a serpent and receiving a foot massage from his consort Lakshmi. This image suggests that massage is a favorite pastime even of Lord Vishnu.

In the Indian home, massage can help maintain a loving relationship between husband and wife. After this kind of soothing relaxation, it is easier to share and give more love. Coming home from a long day of work in the outside world, the husband can often be found receiving a loving massage from his wife. This type of massage is not usually done with oil—the muscles are just gently squeezed and rubbed. Even the older family members receive a form of massage as grandchildren press against their bodies in play.

Ceremonial massages are also practiced in India. Massage before marriage is one of the few ceremonial massages in the Hindu tradition that is compulsory even today. This is because it lends a glow to the skin and relaxes the couple, making them look fresh and shiny. For the groom, the massage can also provide an increase in virility and psychic strength. Because the massage is done with natural herbs and oils, it makes the bride more fragrant and beautiful.

Another traditionally compulsory massage is the one given daily to the new mother during the forty days following birth. Traditionally this is the time for a woman's complete body purification, after which she can return to performing her daily worship or household chores.

The ancient science of Indian massage was described by Valmiki, the first poet of the Sanskrit language, in his epic poem the Ramayana. The Persian and Greek (Unani) systems of massage strongly influenced the basic forms of massage developed in the West. Many common elements can be found between Persian and Greek massage and Ayurvedic massage; Unani massage utilizes the three humors as well as similar herbs, spices, herbal formulas, and oils. Their ways of living happy and healthy lives, common among the three cultures, extended to a similarity in martial art styles and massage methods. Because of this cross-fertilization, the strokes of the Eastern and Western systems seem strangely similar.

Massage is growing in popularity in the West in response to an increase in the stresses and strains in this world of greed and competition. With the increase in pollution—of air, water, and sound—our nerves are constantly being agitated. Our glands are constantly being overstimulated by the use of preservatives. With the increase in packaged and precooked foods, more chemicals are permeating our bodies on a cellular level. Fresh milk from the farmer's cow is like a dream, and processed milk is loaded with chemicals. Grains and vegetables grown without synthetic fertilizers are almost extinct. To maintain good health, we have no choice but to learn ways to help flush these toxins from our systems as regularly as they are ingested. Massage is one of the few remedies known for doing this. Regular massage, along with ingesting organically grown foods and pure water and performing exercises in natural sunlight in an unpolluted environment, can prove extremely beneficial.

Massage works on both the physical and mental levels. Physically, it helps all systems of the body—the immune, respiratory, nervous, endocrine, circulatory, muscular, skeletal, digestive, and lymphatic. Mentally, it helps the mind relax. This is especially true when one has good feelings toward the practitioner. Generally, massage assists the body in self-healing. By easily and naturally concentrating on the body part being worked, the recipient can transmit positive life-giving energy to himself whenever and wherever needed. Massage can make the mind stop wandering and give perfect relaxation, providing it is not the kind of massage that hurts. Self-massage offers all of the above-mentioned benefits except the soothing touch of another, which itself can yield miracles.

Chapter One

Introduction to Massage

MASSAGE AS A DAILY PRACTICE

Massaging the body daily for thirty to forty-five minutes before bathing can improve one's health and vigor. By rubbing the skin the body becomes heated, which in turn thins the blood and helps it circulate through the system. Since this heat also opens the pores, it is important not to take a bath until the body has absorbed the oils and cooled to at least normal room temperature. This usually takes thirty minutes to one hour from the completion of the massage.

Massage is essential for all people in all stages of life—infants, householders, elderly, handicapped, infirm, or bodybuilders. For people unable to exercise, massage is an excellent alternative for enhancing the growth and development of the body. And for the young and energetic people who are busy practicing the martial arts, massage is a must. The muscular strain acquired during workout sessions can only be relieved by massage. It refreshes the muscles, bringing them back to their original shape.

For people suffering from sleeplessness or disturbed sleep, receiving a massage, or even self-massage, is essential. Foot massage, which is good for the entire system, is especially recommended for those suffering from fatigue. According to Charaka, the author of the well-known Ayurvedic text *Charaka Samhita*, people with insomnia should be given a head massage before retiring. For even greater results, he recommends a combination foot, spine, and head massage.

MASSAGE AS AN EXERCISE

Massage should be an exercise for the practitioner. Since a good massage calls for vital energy or pranic force, one who gives a massage has to breathe deeply and slowly. Attention should be paid to not becoming breathless, as this puts a strain on the heart and can dilate the cardiac muscles. The practitioner should be able to control his or her breathing, relaxing between strokes to inhale deeply. A good massage should generate a sweat in the practitioner, which is beneficial.

When given as a form of exercise, the strokes are hard. By applying bearable kneading and rubbing pressure, the practitioner's pranic force and muscle power are strengthened.

MASSAGE AS RELAXATION

If carried out in a gentle manner, massage is an excellent relaxation technique. The practitioner's hands should be warmed by rubbing them against each other, then lubricated with a fragrant oil to avoid causing friction, irritation, or uneasiness. Massage of the spine, feet and arms, shoulders, and head can become an enjoyable experience for anyone and everyone. Massage of the pressure points (the marmas) relaxes the body instantly. If the practitioner is not relaxed, then the person receiving the massage cannot fully relax. Relaxation massage should reduce the speed of the breath and mind in both parties.

With aging comes the gradual loss of agility and quickness. The physical and mental strain that accumulates each day while one performs unnatural activities causes weakness in the nerves and impairs circulation of the vital life fluids. Tension, constant worry, dissatisfaction, greed, and anxiety are bound to affect the organism. These enemies bring on premature aging. To avoid this problem, and to reduce the stress on the body and mind, relaxation is a must. While yoga postures and deep-breathing exercises ensure relaxation, massage offers even more benefits. This is because massage employs, in addition to muscular stimulation, the miracle of touch and fragrant oils prepared from rejuvenating herbs. In sum, massage can stop premature aging, reduce wrinkles, tone muscles, and restore agility to joints. It lends a smooth texture to the skin, strengthens the nerves and the immune system, and helps the body retain its proper shape and elasticity. Regularity is key in obtaining the maximum benefit from massage.

HEALING BENEFITS OF MASSAGE

Life in modern times has become very luxurious in some ways. Most people who live in towns and cities do little physical labor. The demands of their jobs don't allow them to participate in activities that make their muscles work. Coupled with not enjoying fresh air, naturally grown foods, or sunlight, their systems become imbalanced. Constant worry and stress increase the accumulation of toxins in their system. The best, easiest, and most natural remedy for all of these problems is massage.

If the entire body cannot be massaged, at least a foot massage should be done each night before going to sleep. The head should be given a massage once or twice a week, or every third day.

Regular massage, given even once or twice a week, prevents the development of many skin disorders such as eczema, blisters, scabies, and seborrhea. It also increases stamina, patience, self-confidence, forbearance, wit and intelligence, sexual vitality, and physical beauty.

Massage is therapeutically used for neurasthenia, headaches, insomnia, gout, polio, obesity, arthritis, blood pressure irregularities, asthma, and mental disorders. Massage increases the body's production of white blood corpuscles and antibodies, which provide resistance against viruses and diseases produced by infections. It helps the defense mechanisms of the body and strengthens the immune system. Massage also increases the body's ability to adapt to sudden changes in temperature and atmospheric pressure, as well as to other environmental changes.

Regular massage helps balance the three body humors, known in Ayurveda as doshas: *vata* (wind), *pitta* (bile), and *kapha* (mucus). It also establishes balance among the three fundamental principles—*sattva*, *rajas*, and *tamas*. (These principles will be discussed later in the text.)

When massage is adopted as a daily practice, it offers many pleasurable benefits. Body heat and vitality increase as the circulatory and respiratory systems open to provide fresh oxygen and vital energy in the form of nutrient material. Simultaneously, waste gases and toxins are flushed from the system.

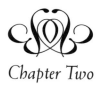

Chapter Two

Ayurvedic Principles of Massage

The Sanskrit term Ayurveda is a combination of two words: *ayu* (life) and *veda* (knowledge). The literal translation of Ayurveda is "knowledge of life" or "right living." Its principles are universally applicable. Those who wish to live happy, healthy, and inspired lives can benefit from the wisdom Ayurveda holds.

Ayurvedic knowledge is grounded in the Vedic scriptures, which date back to 3000 B.C. According to the Vedas, life is seen as an evolution of the creative principle, Prakriti, and the formless and attributeless nonbeing, Purusha. While Prakriti is the Shakti, or Divine Mother, Purusha is the Father principle, which is unchanging. Prakriti creates all forms in the universe. In their primary states all forms contain the three *gunas*, or principles (sattva, rajas, and tamas), in perfect balance. When the gunas start to interact, the balance is disturbed. In an attempt to restore this balance, activity begins. This action creates currents of energy, and space, or *Akash*, is generated. From Akash comes Air, from Air comes Fire, then come Water and Earth. Simultaneously, during this process of creation, three fields are created: the mental (conscious) field, created by Sattva; the power field, created by Rajas; and the material field, created by Tamas. The five elements belong to the material field and are the building blocks of the body.

Tridosha and the Five Elements

The *tridosha* theory—vata (wind), pitta (bile), and kapha (mucus)—is unique to Ayurveda. These three doshas constitute the chemical nature of every living organism; they are created by the five elements in the following way. The elements of ether and air *(akash* and *vayu)* form the vata temperament; fire and water *(agni* and *apah)* form the pitta temperament; water and earth *(apah* and *prithvi)* form the kapha temperament. Within the body, bones, flesh, skin, nerves, and hair belong to the earth element. Semen, blood, fat, urine, mucus, saliva, and lymphatic fluid belong to the water element. Hunger, thirst, body temperature, sleep, lethargy, intelligence, anger, hate, jealously, and radiance belong to the fire element. All movements—breathing, natural urges, sensory and motor function, secretions and excretions, and transformation of tissues—belong to the air element. Love, enmity, shyness, fear, and attachment are qualities identified with the akash or ether.

Each individual's temperament, or *prakriti,* is determined at the time of conception and is unchangeable during one's lifetime. The chemical environment of the ovum fertilization plays an important role in establishing the psychosomatic nature of an individual. By the interaction of the individual and the environment, imbalances in one's prakriti occur. These imbalances are referred to as one's *vikriti.*

TYPES OF TEMPERAMENTS

According to Ayurveda, one (and often two) of these seven temperaments can be found in all living organisms:

1. Vata (wind-dominated)

2. Pitta (bile-dominated)

3. Kapha (mucus-dominated)

4. Kapha-pitta (dominated by a combination of wind and bile)

5. Pitta-kapha (dominated by bile and mucus)

6. Vata-kapha (dominated by wind and mucus)

7. Vata-pitta-kapha (dominated equally by all three doshas)

Additionally, when the varying proportions of vata, pitta, and kapha are considered, an innumerable variety of temperaments exist.

Through these doshas the human organism accepts environmental changes and receives energy from food. The workings of all three doshas is most concentrated in the region between the heart and the navel. It is here that the doshas ceaselessly interact, carrying on the body's task of self-preservation and growth. Any disturbance in one dosha immediately creates an imbalance in the body and interrupts the discharge of waste material.

A harmonious balance of all three doshas is essential for the maintenance of physical and mental well-being. Disturbance of any one dosha creates disease and disorder within the organism. Because of the crucial role the tridoshic system plays in the regulation, preservation, and growth of our bodies, it must be studied by every Ayurvedic massage practitioner. Examination of the radial pulse is essential for determining a person's vikriti and must be learned by the massage practitioner (see page 17). To select the appropriate oil, it is necessary to know which dosha is aggravated. (See chapter 3 for a discussion of doshas and oils.)

The state of one's body chemistry varies according to such factors as place, climate, and diet. Underlying these factors, which can vary daily, there exists one's prakriti—a basic chemical blueprint on which the organism has been constructed. This genetic code dictates many aspects of an individual, such as his or her likes and dislikes, choices of food, and preferences regarding taste, flavor, and temperature. While Vata and Pitta types can receive enormous benefit from oil massage, Kapha types should concentrate on dry massage or massage with medicated oil made especially for their type.

Vata

People of the vata temperament—those dominated by vayu (wind)—sleep little, walk fast, and talk too much. Their bodies are dry, and their hair is thin, sparse, and brittle. They have restless minds and their feelings roam from place to place almost continuously. They dislike cold and cold items, have weak memories, and leave many sentences incomplete because their minds switch abruptly from one thought to another. They are lovers of sexual and sensual enjoyments and are especially fond of sweet-, sour-, hot-, and pungent-tasting foods. They eat too much or too little, and produce sounds while drinking water. Basically, Vata individuals are unpredictable and insecure. They spend money quickly and tend to remain poor. The life span of the Vata individual is relatively short. Vata people dream of dwelling on mountains, in trees, and in the air, and of flying without mechanical aids. The Vata body is tall and thin, with knees that are knobby and weak. The pulse is feeble and moves like a snake.

When wind (vayu) is disturbed it is characterized by the following types of conditions: excessive thirst; shaking; dryness; roughness; redness of skin; pain; asthma; cough; ailments of ears, nose, and throat; circulatory troubles; urinary ailments; and constipation.

If vata (vayu) continues to increase, it creates roughness of the voice, throbbing sensations, and a desire for heat; it darkens the complexion and leads to weakness. If vayu decreases, it produces uneasiness and sometimes unconsciousness.

Pitta

People of the pitta temperament—those dominated by bile—have angry dispositions and sweat profusely; they are also learned, brave, and proud. Their hair is soft, oily, and yellow, and becomes white or gray at an early age. They are lovers of flowers and aromas. People of good character with a spiritual outlook, they are kind, courageous, and will save even their worst enemies. Pittas do not follow the religion in vogue, and their attachment to the opposite sex is minimal. They are lovers of sweet-, bitter-, and astringent-tasting foods, and are especially fond of cold drinks. They are jealous by nature and frequent the bathroom often. Their color is fair and body temperature is hot. Their joints and muscles are loose and their virility and sexual desire not strong. Their eyes are red, and get more red with anger, intoxication, or exposure to sunlight. Their life span is average. Pittas have soft, oily, and warm skin. They are aggressive and avoid disturbances or frequenting places where there are likely to be quarrels. They dream of fire, falling stars, lightning, sun, moon, shining objects, and poisonous plants. They spend money on luxuries and devise their own methods of earning a living.

When pitta is disturbed it is characterized by burning sensations, acidity, thirst, irritability, redness of the eyes, indigestion, heat in the chest and stomach, skin diseases, defective vision, perspiration, and hysteria.

If pitta continues to increase, it produces aggravated burning sensations, preferences for cool and cooling foods, yellow eyes and complexion, yellow stools and urine, insomnia, fainting, and diminished functioning of the sense organs. If pitta decreases, it produces a dull complexion and diminished body heat.

Kapha

People of the kapha temperament—those dominated by mucus—have a forgiving disposition and a great deal of virility. Their bodies are well constructed and padded, sometimes with too much fat. The Kapha mind is stable; they are sober people by nature. Their faces are moonlike and their joints are well constructed, strong, smooth, and deep. The body has the color of brass, gold, or a lotus flower, with long hands and a broad and strong chest. They are attractive, with broad foreheads and tender bodies. Kaphas have strong hair that is oily, dense, thick, and wavy. They are not disturbed by hunger, thirst, pain, interruptions, or noise. Wise and fond of order, Kaphas honor their word. They follow the principles and practices of right living; they are soft-spoken but hold on to hostility toward their enemies for a long time. Kaphas are great lovers of sexual pleasures. They are industrious, humble, and slow. They love bitter-, astringent-, sharp-, and dry-tasting foods and have a tendency to sleep soundly and for a long time. They dream of rivers, ponds, oceans, lakes, waterbirds, and lotuses.

When kapha is disturbed, it is characterized by heaviness, drowsiness, numbness, itching, nausea, anorexia, dyspepsia, loss of memory, white urine and stool, heaviness and rigidity in the joints, and a feeling of aging. Often a sweet taste in the mouth is experienced.

If kapha continues to increase, it produces an increased heaviness in the limbs, cold sensations, excessive sleep, looseness of joints, drowsiness, and a pallid complexion. If kapha decreases, it produces dryness, an internal burning sensation, a feeling of emptiness in the stomach and intestines, thirst, weakness in the joints, general weakness, and insomnia.

BENEFITS OF AYURVEDIC MASSAGE

In Ayurveda, massage is highly praised and recommended as a daily practice. As people follow the daily practice of eating and sleeping, so should they receive massage and discharge waste materials.

Ayurveda believes that pains and aches are caused by obstruction of the flow of vayu (wind) through vayu-carrying vessels, or *siras*. Heat is generated by rubbing, which makes the body airs expand and move. Circulation of vayu in the siras relieves tension and reduces pain. Massage also promotes a deeper and more natural breathing pattern.

Regular massage relaxes the muscles, nerves, bones, and the whole body. It aids the digestive system by maintaining the proper balance and circulation of body gases; it induces deep sleep, increases the appetite, and generally makes life more joyful.

In therapeutic massage, the type of massage administered and the oil used depend on the condition present. According to Vagbhata, the author of a famous treatise on Ayurveda called *Ashtanga Hridaya*, those who wish to have health and happiness should massage the body and use oils according to the season. Fragrant and health-giving organic oils are best.

According to another key scripture on Ayurveda, the *Sushruta Samhita*, oil, ghee,* or any other lubricant—depending on the body type, the atmosphere, and the season—should be used for massage. For those suffering from a wind (vata) disorder, massage is the only remedy. Generally, massage of especially tense areas should not be done without a proper lubricant. Areas that are painful should be massaged until some relief is obtained.

The role of massage in sexual enjoyment is emphasized by Vatsyayana, the author of the well-known treatise on sex, the *Kama Sutra*. In the Bhavishya Purana, a religious scripture, the importance of massage between husband and

---

* Ghee is sometimes referred to as clarified butter, which is made by heating butter gently until the milk solids settle at the bottom of the pan. The clarified butter is then ladled off the top and used for cooking. In India, ghee is traditionally made by churning yogurt into butter, which is then melted to make ghee. Both clarified butter and traditional ghee are appropriate for massage.

wife is described in detail. The scripture advises that the wife should be an expert in the art of giving massage. It recommends that massage of the waist region be done gently and slowly, and that the face and neck should be massaged a little harder, with bearable pressure. The head and feet should be massaged the hardest, and for a longer period of time. Those body parts having less flesh, thin musculature (such as the navel area), and certain pressure points below the navel and around the heart, face, and cheeks should be massaged gently. If the husband starts to doze off, rubbing and patting can be done; when he falls asleep, the massage should be stopped. On the body parts that have hair, the massage should be done in the direction of hair growth.

The following benefits of massage can be found in the *Ashtanga Hridaya* of Vagbhata.

Removes Old Age (Jarahar)

In Ayurveda, massage is described as jarahar, the remover of old age, because it provides nourishment to the seven constituents, or *dhatus*, of the human body:

1. Rasa (fluids, hormones, lymph)

2. Rakta (blood)

3. Mansa (flesh, muscles, and cutis)

4. Medha (fat)

5. Asthi (bones and teeth)

6. Majja (marrow)

7. Shukra (semen, ojas)

By rubbing, squeezing, and pressing the musculature and by manipulating the pressure points, circulation of blood, lymph, and hormones is enhanced. This in turn strengthens the nervous and immune systems, thus delaying old age. The use of oil on the spine, feet, hands, and head increases virility and vitality.

Removes Fatigue (Shram Har)

Fatigue is caused by either physical or mental strain, or both. It can also come from overworking a particular muscle or muscle group, or doing work one does not normally do. When one does not feel emotionally involved in a job or does not like it, his or her body fatigues quickly. Fatigue can also be a product of accumulated toxins. The massage prescribed depends on the type of fatigue present.

For fatigue caused by mental strain, a head massage with a fragrant oil is ideal. A few drops of sandalwood oil added to the base massage oil helps relieve mental strain. To remove heat from the head area, apply a mix of 10 drops of coriander oil and 2 tablespoons of almond or sesame oil.

For fatigue caused by physically straining the muscles of a limb, add a pinch of salt to some warm water and immerse the limb in it. Massage it with a squeezing motion. If immersion is too difficult, soak a towel in the hot salted water and apply it to the painful area. This method is mostly used on the shoulder and waist region. (Alternating hot and cold towel compresses may be used as well.) Gently squeezing, rubbing, and patting muscles removes fatigue. After water treatment, oil should be applied until release is felt. A half cup of mustard, almond, coconut, or sesame oil to which a few drops of lavender, wintergreen, or spirit of camphor oil are added helps to remove strain from aching muscles.*

To remove fatigue caused by an accumulation of toxins, you may use an oil that is heating—one that produces a burning sensation on application. This will excite the sweat glands and stimulate the body to release the toxins through sweat. Some heating oils are wintergreen, mint, mustard oil, eucalyptus oil, and oils made from garlic, asafoetida, or fenugreek seeds.

Removes Excess Wind (Vata Har)

The following practices, emotions, or food excesses increase the dosha of wind (vata) and can cause pain in the muscles and joints: constant strain on the nervous system; anxiety; sexual indulgence after eating; eating food stored for more than eight hours after cooking; sleeping during the day; suppression of hunger; fasting; voluntarily repressing any natural urge of the body; cracking of the joints; sexual intercourse during menstruation; oral sex; fear; nervousness; excessive talking; excessive use of pungent, astringent, or extremely bitter foods. Foods such as beans, lentils, soybeans, broccoli, cabbage, and cauliflower, when used in excess, produce more vayu and the ailments caused by aggravated wind. Rheumatism and sciatica are two of the most common ailments caused by aggravated wind.

The seat of vata diseases is the large intestines. Colon therapy or water purification, done as soon as the ailment is detected, and regular massage with oil are the only remedy. The *Sushruta Samhita* strongly recommends oil massage for vata disorders. In Ayurveda, *mahanarayana* oil, a medicinal oil expressed from various plants, is often recommended for rheumatic pains and sciatica.

Sesame *(til)* oil prepared with the following herbs and spices is recommended for vata disorders. Cook a clove of garlic in preheated oil until it turns black. Add 1 teaspoon fenugreek seeds and cook 2 minutes. Stir in a pinch of asafoetida

---

* People with sensitive skin should not use this formula. Instead, they should mix a few drops of sandalwood oil with any other base oil that is compatible with their dosha.

and heat for 3 minutes more. Finally stir in 1 teaspoon oregano seeds and heat until they turn brown. Strain the oil and store in a container with a tight-fitting lid.* To lend a nice scent, a few drops of lavender, mint, or wintergreen oil (or all three) may be added.

Improves Eyesight (Drishti Prasad Kar)

According to Ayurveda, massage can improve one's eyesight. Eyes derive their primary energy from the fire element. Disorders of the stomach in which the digestive fire is high create most eye ailments, although low fire can also cause disturbances. Constant constipation (caused by low fire), indigestion and acidity in the stomach, and aggravation of pitta (bile) impair one's vision. Massage of the navel area in a clockwise direction with coconut or sesame oil (depending on one's constitution) before retiring improves eyesight. People who have weak vision or who suffer from eye diseases should massage their feet, especially between the big toe and second toe. They should also have their spine, neck, and head massaged regularly with oil. (See Oils for Head Massage, page 90, for oil beneficial to the head.)

There are five subtypes of pitta and the one found in the eyes is called *alochaka pitta*. It aids vision, balances heat in the eye tissues and muscles, and is responsible for regulating light input. Massage of the head and the big toes helps to regulate this fiery element. Eyes have a healing system all their own. Through the chemicals present in tears, the eyes become revitalized. Tears produced by the application of eye remedies such as *surma* and *kajal* (see page 134–35), ghee, honey, or onion juice are cleansing, rejuvenating, and healthy for the eyes. Tears produced by sorrow, anger, disgust, and sickness are sour and can damage the eyes. The practice of *tratak* (gazing into a flame until tears come) is a healthy exercise for the eyes.

Massage of the temples with oil or ghee can improve eyesight as well. The practices of *jala neti* (taking water in through the nose) and massaging the inner walls of the nose deeply and gently with ghee are also quite helpful for the eyes.

Strengthens the Body (Pushti Kar)

Rubbing with massage oil and pressing, with or without oil, is beneficial for the body. It increases circulation and movement of the vital life fluids while at the same time helping to enhance and circulate pranic energy. By kneading and pressing the muscles, accumulated toxins are encouraged to leave the body; in exchange the cells fill with nutrient material and prana. The body and the immune system become strong, and stamina, vitality, and virility increase.

---

* Adding mustard or fenugreek seeds, as well as dry or green fenugreek leaves, to food is also helpful in vata disorders.

Increases Longevity (Ayus Kar)

Massage creates an electrochemical balance in the body. When the body's immune system becomes strong and toxins are eliminated, longevity is naturally increased. Since an increase in acidity reduces life span, our blood chemistry should always be more alkaline than acidic. Anxiety and stress wear out the system and increase acidity in the system. Balancing the three doshas increases our life span. The use of rejuvenating oils, prepared with herbs and spices, enhances the life force of the body. These oils are absorbed by the skin and digested into the body, with the help of a subtype of pitta called *bhrajaka pitta.* The absorbed oil protects the skin from dehydration and helps it retain the necessary amount of surface moisture. This moisture helps the electromagnetic energy of the earth to react with the electromagnetic field of the body. In old age this moisture diminishes, the skin becomes dry, and the body does not get enough energy from the environment. Through massage an electrochemical balance can be maintained, which results in health and long life.

Induces Sleep and Dreams (Swapna Kar)

Massage in general, and head massage in particular, is an effective device for inducing sleep. Gentle rubbing, patting, and pressing of the body, especially the feet, help soothe the wandering mind. People suffering from insomnia or disturbed sleep should massage their body before retiring. (Of course, it is better if the massage is given by someone else.) Coconut or sesame oil should be used for the body and feet, and *kaddu* oil, extracted from the pumpkin seed, should be used for the head.

Strengthens the Skin (Twak Dridh Kar)

Massage with oil makes the skin feel smooth and gives it a glow. Regular application strengthens the skin and removes dryness, the first sign of disturbed wind (vata) in the body. Individuals whose prakriti, or constitutional type, is vata have dry and rough skin; for them, oil massage is a must. For those people whose prakriti is either pitta or kapha, and thus who naturally have oily skin, oil massage is the only remedy when wind is aggravated and dryness of the skin appears. Dryness of the skin can also be caused by meditation, mental work, anxiety and worry, and living in centrally heated homes. For people who get dry skin from cold outside air, central heating compounds their problem.

Just as fire is hot by nature, wind by nature is cold and dry. Since people with a vata temperament tend to have closed hair follicles; for them it is appropriate to apply the oil *against* the direction of the body hair to help open these follicles. Once the oil has been applied, the practitioner can then massage in the direction of the body hair. The skin of vata-dominated people absorbs more oil than

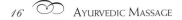
that of other types. Skin, like a mirror, reflects the state of the physical body. Wheat germ oil mixed with almond oil is especially good for strengthening the skin. Oils provide natural nourishment to the skin, which gets digested by the bhrajaka pitta.

Aids Resistance to Disharmony and Disease
(Klesh Sahattwa)

Rubbing the body with bearable pressure helps make it more resistant to disease. Massage stimulates the production of antibodies and strengthens the seven vital components of the body, the dhatus (see page 12). The strength that comes from the dhatus gives the powers of tolerance, forbearance, and patience; these qualities can save one from sorrow, agony, adversity, and anxiety. Antibodies strengthen the immune system and oils strengthen the nerves.

Soothes Ailments Caused by Wind and Mucus
(Vata-Kapha Nirodhak)

According to the *Sushruta Samhita,* massage with oil is the only effective remedy for soothing diseases caused by aggravated wind (vata); it proves effective as well in diseases caused by aggravated mucus (kapha).

For vata diseases, sesame oil massage is especially recommended; olive, mustard, and almond oil are also prescribed. To help relieve aggravated mucus, congestion of the lungs, or breathlessness, massage of the chest and rib cage region with wintergreen, eucalyptus, mustard, almond, or mint oil is recommended; a mixture of wintergreen, eucalyptus, and almond or mustard oil may also be used. When both wind (vata) and mucus (kapha) are aggravated, the following special garlic/mustard oil mixture is quite effective. Heat $1/4$ cup mustard oil over high heat; when it begins to boil, add 2 medium garlic cloves (peeled) and cook until they turn dark brown. Strain and store. For another good wind (vata) and mucus (kapha) oil mixture, add 5 drops each of wintergreen, mint, and eucalyptus to $1/2$ cup of almond or mustard oil. For easing breathlessness caused by aggravated vata and kapha, a combination of almond and lavender oil can be beneficial. Also, after massage the recipient can inhale the steam from a few drops of eucalyptus oil placed in hot water, taking care to avoid exposure to cold air.

Improves the Color and Texture of the Skin
(Mrija Varn Bal Prad)

Rubbing oil into the skin improves the texture of the skin, gives it a healthy glow, and makes it strong. To nourish the skin and protect it from numerous ailments, add 1 teaspoon turmeric to ¼ cup each of wheat germ, almond, sesame, and coconut oil; strain and cover. To avoid getting a yellow stain on your clothing after massage, add to this mixture an equal amount of sesame or coconut oil, and take a bath after the massage (wait at least 30 minutes to 1 hour before bathing).

In sum, Ayurveda contends that massage is man's best friend. It nourishes all seven dhatus, balances the three doshas, cures diseases caused by aggravation or imbalance in the doshas, rejuvenates the system, provides strength and virility, and removes stress and strain. Ayurveda emphasizes the correct use of different oils in massage. They should be used according to the seasons and the requirements of the particular body in question, as determined by pulse diagnosis.

PULSE DIAGNOSIS

Pulse diagnosis is an extremely important tool in Ayurveda. The information it yields is of great help in selecting the appropriate oil. The pulse should not be examined immediately after eating, bathing, exercise, sunbathing, or sitting near heat; nor should it be taken after massage, after sexual intercourse, or when the recipient feels hungry. These activities can render a reading inaccurate. The recipient should be asked to relax before pulse observation.

The practitioner need not learn all the details of pulse examination that an Ayurvedic physician must learn, or even how to take the pulse that indicates a person's chemical nature or constitution at birth (prakriti). One needs only to be able to detect which dosha is dominant at a given time (vikriti). Ideally, pulse examination is done first thing in the morning, after elimination and before eating.

To observe the pulse, the subject should be in a seated position, facing the practitioner. The subject's elbow and wrist should be slightly bent. The practitioner places his or her index, middle, and ring fingers on the wrist of the subject below the thumb side (see fig. 1). The practitioner's fingers should be loose enough to permit the different movements of the throbbing pulse to be felt simultaneously. Observation of the pulse requires total attention and concentration.

If the throbbing under the index finger is the strongest, then vata (wind) pulse is dominant. The rate of this pulse is around 80 to 100 beats per minute. Pitta (bile) dominates if the throbbing under the middle finger is strongest. The rate of this pulse is around 70 to 80 beats per minute. Kapha (mucus) dominates if the throbbing

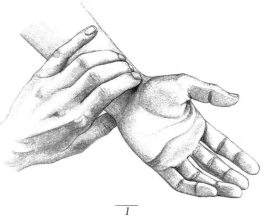

1

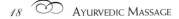

is felt to be strongest under the ring finger. This pulse is the slowest, at 60 to 70 beats per minute. Although the pulse can be checked at six other places in the body,* the practitioner should concentrate only on the radial pulse. Pulse diagnosis should be used by all practitioners, regardless of whether they are performing massage for relaxation or exercise, or for therapeutic reasons.

DOSHAS AND THE SEASONS

As mentioned earlier, environmental factors create imbalances in the doshas. A definite change can be seen in the doshas (wind, bile, mucus) with the change in the seasons and the time of day.

- In spring (March, April, May), kapha (mucus) and pitta (bile) become more dominant in the body chemistry.

- In summer (June, July, August), pitta (bile) dominates.

- In fall (September, October, November), vata (wind) dominates.

- In winter (December, January, February), kapha (mucus) and vata (wind) dominate.

Times of Day

In the early morning hours after sunrise, kapha (mucus) becomes more prominent; at noon, pitta (bile), and in the evening vata (wind) is more dominant.

The cycle repeats itself as follows: after sunset, kapha becomes more prominent; at midnight, pitta dominates; and in the latter part of the night, vata is most prominent. In the life cycles, kapha (mucus) is more dominant in childhood, pitta (bile) during adulthood, and vata (wind) in old age.

THE MARMAS

According to the *Sushruta Samhita,* there are 107 marmas in the human body. Marmas refer to the firm junctures or meeting points of the five organic principles: *mansa* (muscles), *sira* (vessels), *snayu* (ligaments), *asthi* (bones), and *sandhi* (joints). These junctures form the seats of the vital life force or prana. At these junctures, the four classes of sira—nerves, arteries and veins, and lymph—enter the organism to carry nutrients and moisture. These vessels carry vayu; blood, and pitta and kapha when they are dominant; and kapha respectively.

---

* It also can be checked at the following arteries: temporal (just above the temples), carotid (on the inside edge of the sternocleidomastoid muscle, just below the jaw), brachial (inside of the arm, above the elbow), femoral (inside of the thigh, where the leg and pelvis join), posterior tibial (behind the ankle), and dorsalis pedis (on top of the foot).

The *Sushruta Samhita* further classifies marmas according to their relationship to the vital life force. While the amputation of an arm or leg may not prove fatal, a wound to a marma situated in a hand or leg may bring on death.[*] However, the massage practitioner does not need to delve into such detail. Suffice it to know that the marmas sustain the organism. They form the primary seats of the

1. Vayu (wind element);

2. Soma (lunar principle of the organism);

3. Tejas (fiery principle of the organism); and

4. Gunas (sattva, or creation; rajas, or preservation; tamas, or disintegration).

Injury to any one marma can lead to possible deformity, pain, delirium, hallucination, stupor, coma, or death. Injury can also lead to mental illness, as well as loss to one or more dhatus, which are responsible for maintaining the functions of the different organs, systems, and vital parts of the body. While massage in general supplies nourishment to the dhatus, massage of the marmas provides specific help to the dhatus, and thus to the entire organism.

ENERGY TRANSFER AND VIBRATIONS

Massage is an interplay of energies between two bodies. Besides being two human beings, these bodies are also two electromagnetic forces. When we receive or give massage we are not only manipulating muscles, skin, and bones; we are working with energies, both physical and mental. There is a clear interaction between the psyche of the giver and receiver. To understand this, we need to remember one simple law: *Energy flows from a higher level to a lower level.*

The energy transfer process is a simple one. The recipient surrenders to being massaged and allows the body to relax. Defenses drop naturally, allowing the energy of the giver to enter into his or her body and be absorbed. If there is resistance from either party, the massage does not yield many benefits. The receiver needs to allow the giver to work without offering any resistance. This will enable the giver to work with affection and care, to keep his or her vibrational level high, and to not be influenced by personal fantasies or personal thoughts of any kind. Because of engagement in the act of giving, the giver is automatically on a higher level than the recipient. Thus, according to the natural law, the energy is transmitted from the body of the practitioner to the body of the receiver. A fine discharge of electrical energy flows through the fingertips of the practitioner, which the skin of the receiver readily absorbs. Through a fine net-

* For more detailed information on marmas, see *Sushruta Samhita*, volume 2, chapter 6, verses 2–9.

work of subtle nerves called *nadis,* specifically the *pranavaha* and *manovaha nadis,* the pranic energy, as well as the psychic energy, is discharged and absorbed. The marmas play an important role in the absorption of the energy and thus the psychosomatic field of the receiver. Sometimes during massage of the marmas, energy blockages are removed and the receiver experiences emotional changes, such as joy, sorrow, and grief.

If the practitioner does not remain centered during the massage and drifts into the world of fantasies, these fantasies are immediately transmitted through a sympathetic response to the receiver. Similarly, if the practitioner starts thinking about his or her own problems, the receiver also starts feeling problems of a similar nature. Practitioners who have entered massage as a profession and see many people a day can experience energy loss. They should take precautions to restore their energy after each massage. This can be done with the help of nourishing foods, such as fresh milk, nuts, and raisins, and by allowing time for relaxation before and after each session. Lying in the yoga posture called the corpse position *(shavasana)* (see page 51), breathing deeply, and meditating on the sound of one's breath for fifteen minutes will replenish the practitioner's energy. Listening to relaxing music during the massage and relaxation period is also helpful. The practitioner should administer self-massage to his or her fingers and perform slow rhythmic wrist movements before beginning each session.

In India, wrestlers massage each other to engage in the process of energy transfer. They are interested in relaxation, the proper growth of musculature, physical strength, and the tone and elasticity of the body. For this reason, it is easy for them not to fall victim of their fantasies and not to think of personal problems. But those who practice therapeutic massage and concentrate on the sickness of the receiver are susceptible to catching the sickness, if they are not mentally strong and do not have the proper understanding needed to cure the ailment. Study of the construction of the body and knowledge of the marmas and oils all help the practitioner of therapeutic massage concentrate and work with confidence.

The attitude of the practitioner plays an important role in massage. If the goal is only to make money, the practitioner will experience fatigue. If the practitioner enjoys giving massage, understands the responsibility of the job, and treats the profession as a means to serve humanity, the experience will be joyful and less fatiguing. The practitioner should be physically and mentally healthy. A person with soothing vibrations can give a massage with especially beneficial effects. A practitioner should not massage a person that he or she does not approve of at first sight, and vice versa.

In the Ramayana, the famous Indian epic tale about the life of Rama, many battles took place between the warring factions. The weary soldiers were given massages by lovely maidens, sometimes several at a time, and then took a refreshing dip in the river. The maidens, as the author Valmiki describes them, had well-proportioned bodies and eyes that sparkled with light. In India today, however, since the healing powers of touch are known to carry also the potential for sexual arousal, men generally massage men and women massage women. This way the unnecessary waste of energy caused by sensual fantasizing is avoided. To avoid fantasizing when massaging a member of the opposite sex, the practitioner should concentrate on his or her breath, breathing pattern, and heartbeat. If the practitioner works as a vehicle for transferring Divine energy into the body of the receiver, this attitude will change the energy level and the fantasies will not be disturbing.

In family life, it is beneficial for children or young people to massage the older people. If children are taught this art, they can practice it for fun whenever they like. Their energy is pure—they neither fantasize nor suffer from loss of energy.

Professional massage practitioners should learn for themselves what makes them lose energy and what kind of recipients give them inspiration. Only by experience can they learn what to avoid and how to be more useful without feeling exhausted. They can massage members of either sex, if doing so does not present any difficulty. If loss of energy and fatigue is experienced, then fantasizing should be avoided. Just like medical doctors, massage practitioners should develop a neutral attitude toward touching either gender. As a general rule, it is best not to give a massage when one's energy level is low.

In sum, massage is service. Service is the highest *dharma* (religious virtue). A massage practitioner should become a selfless servant and should work without ego.

MASSAGE AND THE LYMPHATIC SYSTEM

Massage works directly and simultaneously with three systems of the human body: the blood/vascular system, the nervous system, and the lymphatic system.

Although it appears to work only with the skin and musculature, massage in fact is transmitted to the vessels of the body. Ayurveda regards the human body as being composed of innumerable channels, or *srotas*, that supply the various tissues of the body. These channels are connected to the marmas and the internal organs. Massage stimulates activity in the channels and enhances circulation of nutrient materials through them to their related organs. According to Ayurveda, these channels are carriers of vayu (wind), pitta (bile), and kapha (mucus), and as such they sustain the human organism. Any obstruction in their flow can generate sickness. Through regular massage, the circulation of vital life fluids can be maintained.

The heart works as a central pumping station, circulating blood charged with nutrient-rich material to the entire body. The nervous system reacts to stimulus and transmits information to the body, allowing it to adjust to the outer environment. The lymphatic system, however, has no main control center. For this reason it is the system most directly influenced by massage and the one most easily damaged by its improper techniques.

In Ayurveda, lymph is considered kaphic in nature. The word *kapha* is usually translated as "mucus" or "phlegm," but its meaning also encompasses lymphatic fluid. *Shlesaka kapha*, a combination of lymph and synovial fluid found in all joints throughout the body, is a white, smooth, cold, sticky, and sweet fluid that acts as a lubricant. It helps reduce the friction within a joint, saving it from wear and tear. Shlesaka kapha also runs along the nervous system, supplying nerves with the power to receive and transmit signals. It helps in the development of antibodies and is thus important for the immune system. The lymphatic system, which works through srotas (vessels) and nodes, restores proteins lost from blood capillaries to the intercellular spaces and transfers absorbed fats and fluids from the intestines to the blood circulatory system.

The lymphatic system is not an independent system. It acts to supplement the blood, and runs parallel to the blood circulatory system. The blood picks up oxygen from the lungs, nutrients from the gastrointestinal tract, and hormones from the endocrine glands. The blood carries these substances to all the tissues of the body, where they diffuse from the capillaries into the tissue fluid. Once in the tissue fluid the nutritive substances are passed on to the cells of that tissue and exchanged for waste. The lymph then picks up materials from the tissue fluid, cleanses them of bacteria, and returns them to the bloodstream. Lymphatic tissue, found in the lymph nodes, the spleen, and the thymus gland, also functions to protect the body from foreign cells and substances. The lymph system, with its army of lymphocytes, phagocytes, and antibody-producing tissues, provides a direct line of defense for the body.

Rather than being a complete circuit, the blood-lymph system is a one-way system: the lymphatic fluid can go into the bloodstream, but blood (or lymph from the blood) cannot enter the lymphatic vessels. The lymph nodes contain no valves and are unevenly distributed in the body. The massage practitioner must remember that the lymph nodes, which produce lymphatic fluid, are located around all the joints of the body. It is possible to stimulate these nodes by a circular rubbing of the joint from all sides. Rubbing deeply into a joint produces heat, enhances circulation, and makes the lymph node secrete its fluid. This in turn will make more protein, glucose, minerals, oxygen, and antibodies available to the blood. The lymph nodes can be excited by other forms of external heat, such as sauna and fomentation (warm and moist local heat).

This complex system can also be stimulated by regular exercise, by compression of the individual lymph nodes or the marmas, and by deep-breathing practices.

When the lymphatic flow is stimulated by means of oil massage, the practitioner can invigorate the blood chemistry and help the body cleanse itself by expelling toxins through sweat and urine. Massage thus can function as a check for the buildup of toxins in the body. Since increased lymphatic flow reduces blood pressure, massage is often prescribed by Ayurvedic doctors for patients suffering from heart trouble and high blood pressure. It is equally helpful for those with low blood pressure because it serves to enhance circulation of the blood and the flow of nutrient materials into the blood.

Chapter Three

Massage Oils

THE ROLE OF OIL IN AYURVEDIC MASSAGE

Ayurvedic doctors as well as Indian wrestlers recommend using oil to receive maximum benefit from massage. Medicated oils are often used by Ayurvedic doctors for curing diseases caused by aggravated vata (wind) and various types of skin disease. A nutrient for the skin, oil contains proteins, carbohydrates, and other essential ingredients that are absorbed through the openings in the hair follicles and assimilated by the bhrajaka pitta. The hair follicles are connected with nerve fibers, which are strengthened by the oil. Oil prevents dryness, increases suppleness, and prevents many of the effects of premature aging. It softens the skin, eliminates friction, disperses heat evenly throughout the body, and provides a smooth luster to the skin. The small amount of oil remaining on the skin after massage, and the shower or bath that follows, provides resistance to the extremes of temperature and pressure in the environment. Application of oil to the navel before going to sleep cures dryness of the whole body. When oil is applied at the junction of the spine and skull, it calms the entire nervous system, strengthens memory, and improves eyesight.

Indian wrestlers never massage their bodies without using oil. It is believed that if the body is rubbed when dry, the friction created generates heat and pain, which aggravates the element of vata (wind) and disturbs the gases in the body. Patting, squeezing, kneading, and gentle pressing (even hard pressing) can be done safely without oil. This can be as beneficial as an oil massage for removing fatigue, stress, nervousness, restlessness, and anxiety. It does not, however, strengthen the nerves and skin, nor does it remove the dryness of the skin. In India, people regularly apply oil to the anus, to prevent itching; to the genitals, to discourage fungal infections; to the nose, to avoid dryness; to the eyes, to clean and strengthen them; to the ears, to clean them; and to the navel, to cure dryness of the body and weak digestive fire. Ayurveda gives much importance to the navel because, through a network of seventy-two thousand subtle nerves (the nadis), it is connected to the entire body. The navel is also the first source of nourishment and life for the fetus. The body needs oil just as any machine used regularly needs oil. It prevents friction, which can quickly ruin costly parts. Oil is both a lubricant and a cleanser, and it conducts heat readily without evaporating. Because of its ability to distribute heat evenly, oil is used as a medium for cooking.

The *Sushruta Samhita* states that the following practices should be adopted by people suffering from vata (wind) diseases:

- Application of *sneha* (lubricant/oil) to an affected area

- Fomentation

- Anointing the entire body

- Oil purgatives

- *Siro vasti* (rubbing oil on the head)

- Oil fumigation[*]

- Gargling with tepid oil

- Using errhines (agents that induce sneezing)

People with vata disorders should also use ghee or clarified butter and oil in cooking, eat saffron and citrus, wash in lukewarm water, have a gentle massage, wear thick garments made of natural fibers (cotton, soft wool, or silk), live in warm rooms, use soft beds, abstain from sex, and bask in the warm glow of a fireplace.

Oil and Dosha Chart

Aggravated (or Dominant) Dosha	Primary Oil
Vata	Sesame[†]
Pitta	Coconut
Kapha	Mustard or olive oil

---

[*] Oil fumigation is a process by which vapors are produced by pouring essential oils onto water that is being continuosly heated. The vapors are then inhaled for beneficial effect.

[†] In cases of vata headaches, wintergreen, eucalyptus, and mint may be mixed with the sesame oil.

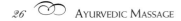

TYPES OF OILS AND THEIR PROPERTIES

Several types of oil may be used for massage, always keeping in mind the aggravated dosha of the client. Cold-pressed oils obtained from the seeds of organically grown plants and vegetables are best. Mineral oils and other substitutes for natural oils are harmful for the metabolic functions of the body. They form a coating or layer on the skin and the cells suffer because they cannot breathe freely. Moisturizers actually increase dryness after a few minutes of use; as well, they most often contain preservatives and are synthetically scented. Commercial oils derived from animal fats present the same problem. In sum, no other lubricant can benefit the skin as well as cold-pressed vegetable seed oils. Easily absorbed, they provide nutrition and help the metabolism. Oils extracted with a wooden oil mill are the best (as compared to oils extracted from mills using metal parts to press the seeds).

Mustard Oil

Mustard oil is a popular oil for massage in India. Wrestlers and bodybuilders prefer it because of its power to relieve the muscle stiffness that comes from wrestling and intense bodybuilding exercises.

Mustard oil is unctuous, bitter, pungent, sharp, light, and heating. Mustard oil destroys diseases caused by vata (wind) and kapha (mucus); it increases pitta (bile) and body heat. A wormicide and fungicide, it cures pain, swelling, and wounds of all kinds. Mustard oil also disinfects and, if used on cuts immediately, stops bleeding. It is readily absorbed when rubbed into the skin, and provides relief for nerves and stiff muscles and ligaments. It removes stiffness in muscles caused by fever and bronchitis, cleanses the blood, and opens the pores. Mustard oil extracted from yellow mustard seeds can be applied to the eyes without any harmful effects. No other oil is as effective and harmless when applied to delicate areas, such as the nose, ear, throat, anus, or genitals. It also can strengthen the skin and enhance pigmentation.

For people with arthritis and gout, Ayurvedic texts recommend massage with a mixture of mustard oil and organic camphor: Slowly heat $^1/_4$ cup of oil with $^3/_{16}$ teaspoon of organic camphor over low heat until dissolved.

An earache that starts suddenly can be cured by placing a few drops of lukewarm mustard oil into the afflicted ear.

For swelling of any kind, massage with warm mustard oil is very beneficial. For quicker results, heat one of the following in 2 tablespoons of oil: a few cloves of garlic, $^1/_2$ teaspoon of asafoetida, or $^1/_2$ teaspoon fenugreek seeds. Cook until black and strain before using. (If the pure gum form of asafoetida is available, use an amount equal to the size of a green pea.)

Massage of the stomach and abdominal region with mustard oil arrests enlargement of the spleen and helps in its cure.

For any kind of dryness, skin irritation, or rash, a massage using mustard oil combined with a little turmeric powder can bring relief. The addition to this mixture of a small amount of organic camphor or spirit of camphor can bring cooling relief and simultaneously remove any itching.

Prolonged and regular use of mustard oil on the hair prevents it from falling out and graying.

People with very sensitive skin may feel irritation when using mustard oil, which may be related to using a poor-quality oil. Most of the mustard oil sold today is made from black mustard seeds, which is acceptable for massage provided it is of high quality. Always look for cold-pressed, fresh oil. The best mustard oil is that which has been extracted from yellow mustard seeds and pressed through a wooden mill but that is a rare find today.

Olive Oil

Olive oil is unctuous, slightly bitter, and heating; it increases pitta (bile) and is nourishing. It contains proteins, minerals, and olein. Olive oil is popular in Middle Eastern countries and the West, where it is used as a medium for cooking and in salad dressings. Some scientific research done in Europe shows that olive oil can work as a preventive against osteomalacia (softening of the bone). It stops infections, has a beneficial effect on the flora of the digestive tract, activates the flow of bile, and stimulates fat metabolism.

Olive oil can be used for massage, although it is stickier and heavier than other massage oils. In India olive oil is rare and costly because it is imported. For this reason it is used only in medicinal massage. Ayurvedic doctors (vaidyas) and Muslim doctors who follow the Greek system of medicine (hakims) prescribe olive oil massage for relief from gout, arthritis, muscular pains, sprains, and polio. It is praised as being hotter and more nourishing than sesame or mustard oil, and as good for the body as almond oil.

Since olive oil is heavy and absorbs solar radiation, massage with it before a sunbath would make the body more receptive to sunlight. Its stickiness and heaviness can be reduced by adding a little sesame oil; a few drops of a fragrant essential oil such as jasmine, rose, or lavender makes it an ideal massage oil. It is especially beneficial to infants, children with weak constitutions, and the elderly. It strengthens the muscles, skin, and nerves; it also cures swelling and enhances pigmentation. It is not good for the hair, however. Whenever olive oil is used for head massage, an herbal shampoo or soap-nut powder (reetha), should be used to wash it out. (Reetha can be found in some health food stores and in Indian groceries.)

Sesame Oil

Sesame is one of the most popular massage oils, especially in western India. A favorite of Ayurvedic doctors, it is used as a base for medicinal oils.

Sesame oil is unctuous, heavy, sweet, bitter, astringent, and heating. It destroys diseases and disorders caused by vata (wind) and increases pitta (bile); it can be used moderately on kapha (mucus) individuals. Because it contains two natural antioxidants—sesamol and sesamoline—sesame oil will keep for a long time without going rancid. It contains minerals, such as iron, phosphorous, magnesium, copper, silicic acid, and calcium, and trace elements. Sesame oil is also rich in linoleic acid; its lecithin content has a beneficial effect on the endocrine glands and especially on the nerves and brain cells. It contains eight essential amino acids that are important for the brain, which may be why it has a history of being used for head massage and for hair oils.

Black sesame seeds are used in all forms of ritual in India, from birth to death, and are offered to the gods through *homa* (fire sacrifice). Each winter in India it is compulsory for everyone to eat an assortment of foods made of sesame seeds for one day.

Oil made from black sesame seeds cures swelling, removes muscular pain and stiffness, strengthens the skin, and nourishes the hair. It cures dry skin, improves skin texture, and prevents premature aging. Used regularly, it improves the shape of the breasts. Massage with oil from black sesame seeds arrests gray hair and restores it to its natural color, increases vitality and semen, and cures gout and arthritis. It absorbs more prana than other vegetable oils. Because sesame oil is neutral and does not irritate the skin like mustard oil can, and because it is not sticky like olive oil, it is the massage oil of preference. Gray sesame seeds are of medium quality, and the white seeds are only good for eating.

Cold-pressed sesame oil is extracted from a mixture of black, gray, and white seeds. Oil from the black sesame seed is more beneficial for the hair than the clear, light yellowish oil extracted from the gray and white seeds. Perfumed sesame oil makes the hair gray earlier.

Coconut Oil

Coconut oil, used as a base in many cosmetics and soaps, is also a popular oil for massage. Commonly found in tropical and subtropical coastal areas, coconut oil forms 8 percent of the oil and fat supply of the world. Because it solidifies easily, this oil is easy to transport.

Coconut oil is sweet, relatively light, unctuous, and cooling. It is suitable for pitta-dominated people. It cures skin conditions, such as skin rashes, burns, swellings, sores, eczema, and fungal infections; it is commonly used on burns and cuts because of its antiseptic qualities. This oil contains minerals, proteins, carbohydrates, and highly saturated glycerides of lauric, palmitic, and stearic acid. It cures swelling when used orally or added uncooked to salads. In northern India, coconut oil is a favorite among women because it makes the hair healthy, shiny, and long. It can also be used to soothe and cool people whose heads are hot.

When used as a food this oil increases kapha (mucus) unless it is cooked with certain spices. It can, however, be used safely by mucus-dominated people as a massage oil. It is suitable for people living in hot climates. Those who like mustard oil for massage but find it to be a skin irritant can use a mixture of 2 parts coconut oil to 1 part mustard oil.

Massage with coconut oil subdues the body heat that accompanies sexual excitement. Men massaged with it regularly will find that it increases vitality and semen and stops premature ejaculation. Coconut oil is readily absorbed by the skin and improves its texture. Being a relatively light oil, it does not form a coating on the skin. It allows the body to absorb more prana from the atmosphere, in the form of oxygen, negative ions, and solar radiation. For this reason it is good to use as a suntan oil. Placed in a blue glass bottle in the sun for forty days, this oil is capable of curing most burns and so is good to have in the kitchen. If this sun-cured oil is applied to the scalp, palms, and soles, it can reduce fevers. In India coconuts are considered a holy fruit with many healing qualities.

Almond Oil

While almond oil is a good massage oil, it is also costly. For this reason, its use in India as a massage oil is restricted to infants, invalids, and the elderly. Almond oil is sweet, unctuous, heavy, and suitable for kapha-dominated people since it is heating. It contains proteins, minerals, and olein, much like olive oil. It has no chlorophyll but does contain small amounts of linoleic acid, glycerides, saccharose, and asparagin. If placed in an orange glass bottle in the sun for forty days, this oil gives joy, removes pessimism and anxiety, and purifies the blood. Because of its healthy, rejuvenating qualities, sun-cured almond oil is taken with milk as a tonic by Indian wrestlers. It improves their capacity to hold the breath and makes their bodies strong.

When used for massage, almond oil is excellent for muscles and ligaments, cures burning of the skin, increases semen and vitality in men, and cures swelling and dryness of all types. As a hair tonic, it not only cures dryness of the scalp and dandruff, but is also good for the brain.

Castor Oil

Castor oil is sweet, bitter, and astringent as well as heating, heavy, and oily. It is suitable for vata-dominated people. It relieves dry skin and improves the complexion when used externally. Castor oil has healing properties and a nourishing, alkaline effect on the body. It penetrates deeply, into the protective layer under the skin. When taken orally, it acts as a purgative; it cures constipation and many abdominal conditions, such as flatulence, colic, and ulcers. It is useful for eliminating toxins in the form of the undigested food mass known as *ama*. Castor oil serves as an aphrodisiac when taken with dates and milk, and increases one's longevity and strength.

Other Oils

Mineral oils are poor substitutes for plant-based oils. They do not get absorbed by the skin but form a layer on top of it. This serves to seal the pores and prevent the skin from breathing and metabolizing properly. If no other oil is available, it may be used for massage providing the recipient takes a bath as soon as the body returns to its normal temperature.

Baby oils generally contain emulsifiers and are synthetically scented. They do not provide any nutritional benefits to the body or hair, except to temporarily remove dryness. Most baby oils today contain paraffin oil, which in the long run can be harmful. Baby oils should definitely not be used on babies, whose tender skins need nourishing, organic, plant-based oils, free of residues and pesticides. Almond oil, mustard oil, or a mixture of the two helps the growth of muscles and fibers.

OIL FORMULAS AND THEIR USES

The following Ayurvedic formulas have been used over the ages to alleviate dry and rough skin, fatigue, premature aging, and stress and strain. Specific results can be obtained when certain oils are mixed or cooked with particular herbs and spices. Some of these formulas are used by naturopathic physicians today. Essential oils, such as wintergreen, eucalyptus, mint, cinnamon, clove, sandalwood, khus, cedarwood, rose, and camphor, are used in many of the formulas. Additional assistance for certain disease conditions may come from color. Oils acquire different healing qualities according to the color of the glass bottle they are stored in. Green is good for physical healing, and is especially beneficial for vata conditions. If it is not possible to find the proper colored bottle then a clear bottle wrapped in the appropriate colored transparent paper or tissue paper will also work.

OIL FORMULAS FOR THE GENERAL BODY

For women and children

➤ To 4 cups of mustard or sesame oil, add 6 tablespoons sandalwood oil

- To 4 cups of mustard or sesame oil, add 1 cup of almond oil, 2 tablespoons of wheat germ oil, and ¹/₂ cup plus 1¹/₂ tablespoons of sandalwood oil

- To 4 cups of sesame oil, add 3 tablespoons of rose oil

- To 4 cups of sesame oil, add 2 tablespoons of wheat germ oil and 4¹/₂ tablespoons of rose oil

- To 4 cups of sesame oil, add 2 tablespoons each of almond oil, wheat germ oil, and jasmine oil

Store these mixtures in green glass bottles. Keep them outside in the sun during the day and in an open area at night for 40 days.

For men

- To 4 cups of sesame oil, add 2 tablespoons of mustard oil, heated with one of the following: a few cloves of garlic, ¹/₂ teaspoon of asafoetida, ¹/₂ teaspoon of fenugreek seeds, or 1 teaspoon of oregano seeds. (Heat oregano seeds until they turn black.) Filter the mustard oil, then add 3 tablespoons of turmeric and cook until turmeric turns dark brown.* Then add to the sesame oil.

- To 4 cups of sesame oil, add 2 tablespoons of pumpkin seed oil†

Store these mixtures in green glass bottles. Keep them outside in the sun during the day and in an open area at night for 40 days.

For young women

- To 4 cups of black sesame oil, add 2 cups of jasmine oil‡

- To 4 cups of coconut oil, add 1 tablespoon of wheat germ oil and 3 tablespoons of rose oil or 6 tablespoons of sandalwood oil

- To 4 cups of sesame oil, add 2 tablespoons wheat germ oil and 6 tablespoons sandalwood oil

- To 4 cups of sesame oil, add ¹/₄ cup of coconut oil, 2 tablespoons of sunflower oil, and 3 tablespoons of lavender oil

Store these mixtures in green glass bottles. Keep them outside in the sun during the day and in an open area at night for 40 days.

---

* Turmeric strengthens the skin, relieves kapha (mucus) and vata (wind), increases virility, and heals wounds. If mustard oil causes skin irritation, heat the turmeric separately in a little sesame oil and then add it to the larger container.

† This mixture is rejuvenating and strengthening and prevents enlargement of the prostate gland. Pumpkin seeds are a diuretic and a wormicide; they are also high in zinc. Pumpkin oil is cooling and sesame oil is heating. The mixture is vitalizing and nourishes the tissues, muscle fibers, and ligaments.

‡ The jasmine oil referred to in this recipe is oil extracted from sesame seeds that have been treated with jasmine flowers. The jasmine oil sold today in the markets is sesame oil to which the essence of jasmine has been added. The latter only imparts the fragrance; the procedure described for treating the oil with flowers yields true jasmine oil.

For women between forty and fifty

- To 4 cups of black sesame oil, add 2 cups of wheat germ oil and 2 tablespoons of almond oil
- To 4 cups of black sesame oil, add 2 cups of wheat germ oil, 2 tablespoons of olive oil, and either $^1/_2$ cup plus $1^1/_2$ tablespoons of sandalwood or $4^1/_2$ tablespoons of rose oil
- To 4 cups of coconut oil, add 2 cups of black sesame oil, 2 cups of wheat germ oil, 2 tablespoons of almond oil, and 6 tablespoons of lavender oil

Store these mixtures in yellow glass bottles. Keep them outside in the sun during the day and in an open area at night for 40 days.

For women fifty and over

- To 4 cups of black sesame oil, add 2 cups of almond oil, 2 tablespoons of wheat germ oil, and 2 tablespoons of either sandalwood or rose oil
- To 4 cups of black sesame oil, add 2 cups of coconut oil, 2 tablespoons each of almond oil, wheat germ oil, and pumpkin seed oil, and $^1/_2$ cup plus $1^1/_2$ tablespoons of either sandalwood or rose oil

Store these mixtures in orange or red glass bottles. Keep them outside in the sun during the day and in an open area at night for 40 days.

For newlywed men*

- To 4 cups of black sesame oil, add 2 tablespoons of almond oil, 1 tablespoon of wheat germ oil, and 2 teaspoons of cinnamon oil
- To 4 cups of black sesame oil, add 2 tablespoons of olive oil, 1 tablespoon of wheat germ oil, and 1 tablespoon of turmeric powder

Store these mixtures in orange glass bottles. Keep them outside in the sun during the day and in an open area at night for 40 days.

For newlywed women

- To 4 cups of coconut oil, add 2 cups of jasmine oil, 2 tablespoons of almond oil, and 1 tablespoon of wheat germ oil
- To 4 cups of sesame oil, add 2 cups of coconut oil, 2 tablespoons of wheat germ oil, and 3 tablespoons of rose oil

Store these mixtures in clear glass bottles. Keep them outside in the sun during the day and in an open area at night for 40 days.

---

* The bridegroom should take 1 teaspoon of powdered black sesame seeds mixed with $^1/_4$ teaspoon raw sugar. Then he should take the following spiced milk drink. Heat 1 cup of milk and add 5 dates to the pan. Bring to a boil and continue to boil for 3 to 5 minutes. Remove from heat; strain the milk, then mash the dates with a spoon. Combine the milk and the date pulp; add a pinch of saffron before drinking.

OIL FORMULAS ACCORDING TO THE SEASONS

In winter (vata [wind] and kapha [mucus] are dominant)

- To 2 cups of olive oil, add 2 tablespoons of wheat germ oil
- To 2 cups of almond oil, add 2 tablespoons each of wheat germ oil and olive oil
- To 2 cups of sesame oil, add 2 tablespoons each of wheat germ oil and almond oil

In spring (kapha [mucus] and pitta [bile] are dominant)

- To 2 cups of sesame oil, add 2 tablespoons of almond oil
- To 2 cups of sesame oil, add 2 tablespoons of corn or calamus root oil
- To 2 cups of almond oil, add 2 tablespoons each of wheat germ oil and pumpkin seed oil

In summer (pitta [bile] is dominant)

- To 2 cups of coconut oil, add 2 tablespoons of wheat germ oil and 2 tablespoons of sandalwood oil
- To 2 cups of coconut oil, add 2 tablespoons of pumpkin seed oil
- To 2 cups of sesame oil, add 2 tablespoons each of sunflower and pumpkin seed oil

In autumn (vata [wind] is dominant)

- To 2 cups of sesame oil, add 2 tablespoons each of rose oil and castor oil
- To 2 cups of sesame oil, add 2 tablespoons of jasmine oil
- To 2 cups of almond oil, add ¼ cup of sesame oil and 3 tablespoons of sandalwood oil

For cold and rainy days

- Combine 2 tablespoons each of the following five oils: coconut, mustard, sesame, wheat germ, and olive

SPECIAL HOMEMADE OIL FORMULAS

To improve memory

Brahmi (Gotu kola) oil and brahmi-amla (Emblica officinalis) oil are recommended to improve one's memory. Either of these may be purchased ready-made at Indian grocery stores or made fresh according to the following recipes.

Store both these formulas in green, yellow, or orange bottles; these colors are good for memory. Clear glass is also good because it absorbs the full range of color frequencies. If possible keep the bottle outside in sunlight during the day and in an open area at night for 40 days. This will increase the heating effect of the oil and thus enhance its healing power.

Brahmi oil

> 1 cup + 1 tablespoon dried gotu kola leaves
> 4 cups water
> 1 cup + 1 tablespoon sesame oil

Boil gotu kola leaves in water. When three-quarters of the water has evaporated, add the sesame oil. Boil until the remaining water evaporates; as this happens the mixture will take on the consistency of undiluted oil.

Strain the oil and store in a cool, dry place. To 2 cups of brahmi oil add 2 tablespoons of almond oil, which is also good for the brain.

Brahmi-amla oil

> 1 cup + 1 tablespoon dried gotu kola leaves
> 4 cups amla juice extracted from the fresh amla fruit
> 4 cups water
> 2 cups sesame oil
> 2 tablespoons pumpkin seed oil

Boil gotu kola leaves in amla juice and water. When three-quarters of the liquid has evaporated, add the sesame oil. Boil the mixture until the water and juice completely evaporate. As this happens the mixture will take on the consistency of undiluted oil.

Strain the mixture, then add the pumpkin seed oil, which helps forgetfulness.

> ❧ Another formula that strengthens the brain and nervous system, and thus improves memory, can be made by adding $1/4$ cup each of almond and sandalwood oil to 2 cups of sesame oil. This formula can be used as a hair oil by men or women; it helps keep one calm in disturbing circumstances.

To improve circulation

> ❧ To 4 cups of mustard oil, add 1 cup of olive oil and 2 tablespoons each of wintergreen and eucalyptus oil. This mixture provides heat and stimulates the circulation of pranic energy into numb areas or areas of poor circulation.

To relieve chest colds

> ❧ To 2 tablespoons of mustard oil, heated over medium-high heat, add $1/2$ teaspoon of powdered asafoetida or 5 medium-size garlic cloves. Cook for

5 to 7 minutes until the garlic is completely charred or the asafoetida turns dark brown. After the mixture has cooled, filter out the charred garlic and use the remaining seasoned oil for massage. Just before applying, add a pinch of salt. If oil is being prepared for later use, remember to warm oil before administering.

Store this oil in a red glass bottle. If possible keep the bottle outside in sunlight during the day and in an open area at night for 40 days. This will increase its heating effect and thus enhance its healing power.

- *Variation:* 2 teaspoons of fenugreek seeds may be substituted for the garlic or asafoetida. Cook until dark brown. Filter the seeds and apply 2 drops of this oil to each nostril (or each ear) for relief of a runny nose, congestion, or other problems caused by a cold.

- To make another oil remedy that helps relieve chest colds, add 2 teaspoons each of cinnamon and eucalyptus oil to 4 cups of sesame oil. Store in an orange glass bottle and use without heating.

To relieve excess body heat

- Combine 2 tablespoons each of coconut, pumpkin seed, and sunflower oil with 3 teaspoons of essence of rose or 3 tablespoons rose oil. The rose oil mixture is very cooling and cures burns and insect bites. It also removes high fever instantly if massaged on the crown of the head and soles of the feet.

- Combine 2 tablespoons each of coconut and pumpkin seed oil with either 5 teaspoons coriander oil or 3 teaspoons essence of *khus,* the essential oil from kusha grass roots. Khus oil is also good for insect bites and all kinds of burns, including sunburn.

- Combine 2 tablespoons sunflower oil with 1 tablespoon coriander oil. Apply to the head, feet, and navel before retiring.

Store these mixtures in blue glass bottles. Keep them outside in the sun during the day and in an open area at night for 40 days.

To rejuvenate hair

The following formula may be used by men or women. Oiling hair regularly before washing will encourage growth, protect against brittleness, and prevent hair from falling out.

- Combine *bhringaraj* oil, *shikakai* oil, and sesame or coconut oil in equal amounts. Apply to the hair to improve luster and provide nourishment. Leave on overnight and in the morning shampoo with an herbal shampoo or with soap-nut powder, which can be found in Indian groceries. Before shampooing, an amla-powder rinse may be used.*

To relieve insomnia

Kaddu oil, or oil extracted from the pumpkin seed, massaged on the head before going to bed is good for insomnia. *Kahu* oil, which is extracted from the seeds of the kahu tree, is also recommended by Ayurvedic doctors for this condition. The two oils mixed in equal proportion may also be used. If kaddu or kahu oil is unavailable, mix a few drops of sandalwood or rose essential oil to ½ cup of coconut or sesame oil and apply to the head. The oil extracted by means of cold-pressing from a mixture of equal amounts of coriander seeds and black sesame seeds also brings relief from insomnia.

To relieve headaches

Sandalwood oil is ideal for relieving a headache. In India a sandalwood paste is commonly used to cure headaches, and sandalwood is always kept on hand for this purpose. To make a cooling paste, combine a pinch each of organic camphor and saffron with a few drops of sandalwood oil and a few drops of water in a small mortar and pestle, grinding until smooth. Another cooling paste made by grinding cardamom-pod shells with a small amount of water relieves certain types of headaches within a few minutes.

THERAPEUTIC USES OF OILS

- Almond oil: Aids with disorders of the brain and nervous system, burning sensation of the skin, and impure blood; weakness, assists in conditions of old age, and premature aging†

- Babuna (chamomile) oil: Helps muscular pains

- Cream, sweet butter, or ghee: Good for face massage; removes wrinkles

- Camphor oil: Aids bronchitis, rheumatism, sprains, eczema, and skin rash; stops vomiting when taken orally in small amounts; activates the stomach; aids in bile secretion; is a wormicide.

---

* To make this rinse, crush dried pitted amla fruits with a steel or cast-iron mortar and pestle. Strain the powder with a fine sieve or cloth. Soak the powder overnight and strain again. Use only the soaking water as a rinse. If green amla fruits are available, the pulp should be used for washing the hair; otherwise discard the pulp.

† For elderly people or those suffering from general weakness, 1 teaspoon of almond oil mixed in a glass of warm milk with a pinch of saffron gives strength. This combination is also good for those living in cold climates or in the mountains and for people over the age of forty-five.

- Castor oil: Relieves dry skin when used externally; relieves constipation, many abdominal diseases, and rheumatic fever when taken internally; increases pitta (bile) and kapha (mucus); subdues vata (wind)

- Coriander oil: Removes excess body heat

- Clove oil: Aids with teeth and gum problems and bad breath

- Coconut oil: Removes dryness of skin and scalp; soothes skin rashes, sores, and eczema; cures fungal infections

- Kahu oil: Aids insomnia and neurasthenia

- Mustard oil: Destroys diseases caused by vata and kapha and increases pitta and body heat; cures pains, swellings, and wounds of all kinds; is a wormicide

- Olive oil: Helps rheumatism, gout, arthritis, sprains, polio; assists with general muscle, ligament, and nerve weakness

- Pumpkin seed oil: Aids insomnia, anxiety, fever, forgetfulness; rejuvenates; prevents enlargement of the prostate; cures zinc deficiency when used orally; is a wormicide and a diuretic

- Rapeseed oil: Aids bronchitis, rheumatism, sprains, eczema, skin rash; stops vomiting when taken orally in small amounts; activates the stomach; aids in bile secretion; is a wormicide

- Sandalwood oil: Helps impotence, headaches, insomnia, neurasthenia, schizophrenia

- Sesame oil: Destroys disorders of vata; treats swelling, pain, gout, and arthritis; cures dryness and improves the texture of the skin

Ayurvedic Oil Formulas and Their Uses

- Amla oil:* Hair oil

- Bhringaraj oil: For the head and hair; prevents dandruff and dry scalp; soothes pitta

- Brahmi oil: Aids memory and insomnia; for mental strength and sinus problems; stimulates brain tissue; soothes pitta

---

* The amla oil found in Indian markets is not true amla oil. A simple but time-consuming formula for making amla oil is as follows: Soak dried amla fruits in water for 24 hours (the water to fruit ratio is 4:1). Bring misture to a boil and continue boiling until 1/4 of the water remains. Strain the water and add an equal amount of sesame oil. Boil again until no water remains. When cooled, store in a clear glass bottle.

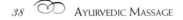
- Brahmi-amla oil: For head massage; use as a hair oil

- Mahanarayana oil: For rheumatism, gout, arthritis, muscular pain, and polio; subdues vata

- Narayan oil (a variation of mahanarayana oil): Good for muscular pain and stiff joints; subdues vata

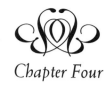

Chapter Four

Preparation for the Massage

Massage is a method of relaxing and strengthening muscles, fibers, tendons, bones, and skin by rubbing, kneading, squeezing, tapping, and sometimes pulling or shaking the tissues. To give a good massage, the practitioner needs to look at the function and form of the musculature. The most effective massage is given by a person who follows the flow of the fluids and natural contours of the body. Working counter to the natural formation of the musculature can create imbalance and disease by introducing tension, damaging fine capillaries, or hurting muscles.

In the Eastern and Western systems of massage, pressing, rubbing, kneading, and squeezing are the same. The sequence of strokes and body parts emphasized in Ayurvedic massage differ from those in the West. Ayurveda places more emphasis on head massage, and oil is placed within the ear. Similarly, massage of the toes and soles of the feet also plays a more prominent role. An Ayurvedic massage is usually somewhat brisk and invigorating and the recipient changes position several times; it also involves the application of pressure to the marmas.

MARMAS

To practice Ayurvedic massage one needs to know the location of the marmas, the pressure points of the body. According to the *Sushruta Samhita*,[*] a marma should be understood as a junction or meeting place of the five organic principles: ligaments, vessels, muscles, bones, and joints. The four types of vessels—

---

[*] *Sushruta Samhita*, Kaviraj Kunjalal Bhishagratna, trans. (Varanasi: Chowkhamba Sanskrit Series Office) p. 178.

nerves, lymph, arteries, and veins—carry vayu (vital energy), pitta, kapha, and blood respectively. These elements enter the marmas to maintain the moisture of the local ligaments, bones, muscles, and joints. In this way the vayu, pitta, kapha, and blood sustain the organism.

Because marmas are the primary seats of vayu, *soma* (the lunar principle), and *tejas* (the fiery principle), as well as of the three fundamental qualities of sattva, rajas, and tamas, they are important for all healers to know about. A massage practitioner should work with the marmas located in the area of the body being massaged to help achieve electrochemical balance in the body. In Ayurveda this is recognized as a balance of sattva, rajas, and tamas. It can also be understood as a balance of the three doshas or constitutional types. By making a gentle circular movement with either the forefinger or middle finger on a marma, toxins can be released and eliminated by the body.*

The practitioner should refer to the following list and to the marma charts on pages 136–41 for identifying marmas in the course of giving a massage.

Classification of Marmas

The 107 marmas in the body can be divided into five classes:

Eleven Mansa Marmas (vulnerable muscle joints)

four Talhridaya	one Guda
four Indravasti	two Stanrohita

Forty-one Sira Marmas (veins or anastomoses)

two Manya dhamni	one Nabhi
two Neela dhamni	two Parshva sandhi
eight Matrika	two Vrihati
four Sringataka	four Lohitaksha
two Apanga	four Urvi
one Sthapni	two Phana
two Apastambha	two Apalapa
one Hridayam	two Stanmula

Twenty-seven Snayu Marmas (vital ligament unions)

four Ani	one Vastih
two Vitapam	four Kshipra
two Kakshadhara	two Ansa
four Kuruchcha	two Vidhuram
four Kurchshirah	two Utkshep

---

* The practitioner's right hand moves clockwise on the marma, and the left hand moves counterclockwise.

Eight Asthi Marmas (bone unions)

two Katika tarunam　　　　　two Ansa phalak

two Nitambatwo　　　　　　two Shankh

Twenty Sandhi Marmas (vulnerable bone joints)

two Janu　　　　　　　　　two Manibandha

two Kurpara　　　　　　　　two Kukundaraya

five Simantakas　　　　　　two Avarta

one Adhipati　　　　　　　　two Krikatika

two Gulpha

Of the 107 total marmas, twenty-two are on the lower extremities (eleven on each leg), twenty-two are on the arms (eleven on each arm), twelve are in the chest and abdomen, fourteen are on the back, and thirty-seven are in the neck and head area.

Names and Location of Marmas

The eleven marmas situated in each leg

1. Kshipra (between the first and second toes)

2. Talhridaya (center of the sole of the foot)

3. Kuruchcha (ball of the foot)

4. Kurchshira (heel and outer margin of the foot)

5. Gulpha (behind both sides of the ankle joint)

6. Indravasti (center of the calf)

7. Janu (the knee joint)

8. Ani (above and lateral to the kneecap)

9. Urvi (middle of the thigh)

10. Lohitaksha (the inguinal region)

11. Vitapam (root of the scrotum)

The eleven marmas found in each arm

1. Kshipra (between the thumb and first finger)

2. Talhridayam (center of the palm)

3. Kuruchcha (above kshipra, root of the thumb)

4. Kurchshira (in the middle of the wrist joint, at the base of the thumb and just below the little finger)

5. Manibandha (the wrist joint)

6. Indravasti (middle of the forearm)

7. Kurpara (inside the elbow joint)

8. Ani (inside the arm, just above the elbow)

9. Urvi (middle of the upper arm)

10. Lohitaksha (axial fold)

11. Kakshadhara (armpit)

The twelve marmas situated in the thorax and abdomen

1. Guda (tip of the tailbone)

2. Vastih (bladder)

3. Nabhi (umbilicus)

4. Hridayam (xiphoid process)

5./6. Stanmula (below the nipple)

7./8. Stanrohita (above the nipple)

9./10. Apalapa (above and to the side of the nipple area)

11./12. Apastambha (between the nipple and the sternum)

The fourteen marmas found in the back

1./2. Katika tarunam (base of the buttocks and the pelvic crest)

3./4. Nitamba (outer iliac crest)

5./6. Kukundaraye (sacroiliac joints)

7./8. Parshva sandhi (above katika tarunam, at the high waist)

9./10. Vrihati (either side of the 10th thoracic vertebra)

11./12. Ansa phalak (shoulder blades)

13./14. Ansa (shoulders)

The thirty-seven marmas located in the neck and head

1./2. Neel dhamni (front of the larynx)

3./4. Manya dhamni (either side of the thyroid)

5. through 12. Eight Siramatrika (arteries on each side of the neck)

13./14. Vidhuram (below the ears)

15./16. Phana (side of each nostril)

17./18. Apanga (outer corner of the eye)

19./20. Avarta (outer side of the eyebrow)

21./22. Shankh (the temple)

23./24. Utkshepa (above the ear)

25. Sthapni (the third eye)

26. through 30. Simantakas (joints of the skull bones)

31./32. Krikatikas (base of skull)

33. through 36. Sringataka (on the soft palate)

37. Adhipati (crown of the head)

THE SPINE

In Sanskrit the spinal cord is called the *meru danda*. Meru is a legendary mountain, supposedly the center of the macrocosm; *danda* translates as "stick." The spine is the center the microcosm, the site of all neuromotor activities of the body. As Mount Meru sustains the body of the macrocosm, our meru danda—our spinal cord—sustains our body.

Constructed like the rattles of a rattlesnake, the spine is capable of making all kinds of serpentlike movements. To maintain its correct shape, the spine must be moved through exercise, yoga, and dance, and should otherwise always be kept erect. Gravity has the least amount of impact on the body when it is erect. In all mental and physical disorders, patients eventually become unable to maintain an erect spine.

Most people are not conscious of the shape of their spine and don't sit erect. This in turn causes many physiological and psychological problems. Generally the spine starts to become deformed after the age of forty-five; this is due in part to the natural aging process and to vitamin deficiencies. Developing a proprioceptive awareness of the spine and its shape and keeping it erect without unnatural supports, such as pillows and backrests, are the first steps toward healthy living.

The vertebrae of the spine create a canal that houses and protects the spinal cord. Connecting with the brainstem and the brain at the cranium, the central nervous system (the brain and spinal cord) is the control center for the whole nervous system complex, which runs throughout the entire body. The motor nerves and the sympathetic and parasympathetic nerves, all relating to the functions of either activity or rest, branch off from the spinal cord and thread through the processes of the vertebrae and the sacrum. From there they branch out to the rest of the body, stimulating muscle and organ tissue and decreasing organ activity. Correct alignment of the spine is therefore key to healthy functioning of the body. The spine is the basis of youth and vigor; the person who maintains its proper shape and stays strong will think properly, act correctly, and live an energetic life.

Proper massage of the spine and vertebral manipulations can cure weak nerves and psychic disorders. Interestingly, in moments of sadness and pessimism the spine becomes loose and collapses. In moments of alertness, inspiration, and joy, the spine automatically becomes erect. The circulation of cerebrospinal fluid, a vital life fluid that is produced in the brain and pumped from the brain down the spinal cord, is critical for maintaining the correct shape of the spine. Since physical exercise, such as walking, yoga, or dance, helps the circulation of this fluid, those who exercise feel inspired and refreshed. This fluid, the nutritive fluid for the nervous system, contains many growth enzymes and is responsible for both physical and mental health. One effective method for maintaining good circulation of this fluid is performing simple spinal twists such as those done in hatha yoga.

When massaging the spine, care must be given to working neither too gently nor too rough. If the massage is too light, mental fantasies are stimulated. If the massage is too rough and unbearable pressure is used, it can have an adverse effect on the nerves and brain. A spinal massage without oil is ineffective. If administered properly—that is, with oil, patience, and the correct amount of pressure—the oil will easily be absorbed by the spine. This routine practice done daily, or at least 3 times a week, will offer lifelong protection against a stiff back and kidney, liver, stomach, lung, or brain disorders.

Massage of the spine is especially important because the spine is the seat of the psychic centers or *chakras*. According to the scriptures of Tantra and Yoga, ancient sciences for achieving higher states of consciousness, the base of the spine is the seat of the dormant spiritual energy called *kundalini*. While the kundalini cannot be awakened through any massage technique, the chakras, which are correlated on the physical plane to the endocrine glands, can be influenced by massage. Spinal massage can induce changes in the body chemistry and release all tension from the body.

If the body is seen as an inverted tree, as described in the Bhagavad Gita, the brain becomes the roots and the spine the trunk. As the erect tree trunk channels the gravitational force through it, so an erect spine supports the body and saves it from being distorted by the pull of gravity.

Duration of Massage

The length of time to give a massage is best determined by the practitioner upon seeing the physical state of the recipient. If the recipient is healthy and interested mainly in relaxation or improved well-being, the massage should not take more than 30 to 45 minutes. If the recipient has tensions, aches, pain, numbness, or poor circulation, special attention should be given to the afflicted areas and the entire massage should take 45 to 60 minutes. People who are physically weak or have a weak constitution should not be massaged more than 30 to 35 minutes. This time should be divided into two or three parts, with rest intervals in between as needed. Slowly and gradually the time can be increased to 45 to 60 minutes. For those who receive massage daily, or who do self-massage, 35 to 40 minutes is sufficient. For infants and newborn babies, 15 minutes is enough. Elderly people who are in good physical health need 1 full hour or more.

DURATION OF MASSAGE

Newborn babies	15 minutes
Infants up to 1 year	15–20 minutes
Children up to 3 years	20–25 minutes
Young people up to 17 years	30–45 minutes
Healthy adults up to 40 years	30–45 minutes
Adults from 40 to 60 years	Depends on their health
Elderly people in good health	60 minutes or more
Invalids	30–35 minutes
People with muscular pain	45–60 minutes

CONTRAINDICATIONS FOR MASSAGE

Do not massage when:

- The person is mucus dominated or has aggravated kapha (mucus), i.e., a cough or cold*

- The person suffers from indigestion, constipation, vomiting, or the first stages of a fever

- The person has just taken a purgative or is involved with the practice of *basti* (enema) as part of a cleansing routine

- The person has just completed a full meal

- The person has just had sexual intercourse

During a whole-body massage, the digestive fire is lowered, which can sometimes aggravate a diseased condition.

---

* A full-body massage should not be given under these conditions, however the chest and rib cage should be massaged with healing oils.

MASSAGE TECHNIQUES

To administer a massage replete with full benefits, one must understand the systematic way of giving a massage. The actual shape of the spine, proper alignment of the vertebrae, location of the pressure points (marmas), and ideal color and texture of the skin must all be studied. It is from the texture of the skin that the practitioner can understand the state of the body and determine its constitutional dosha (prakriti). With a knowledge of the pulses, the practitioner can determine the dosha that is dominant at any given time (vikriti). The practitioner must also know the contraindications for massage, as listed above.

Massage cannot simply be given at any time and in any place. An appropriate environment, location, time, and oil must be selected. The practitioner also needs to be familiar with the psychophysical aspect of the human organism. Not only are skin and muscles involved; so are the delicate art of touching and the many responses to being touched. Touch activates many systems of the body, including the nervous, circulatory, lymphatic, and endocrine systems. At a more subtle level, the practitioner must have a conscious awareness of the role of vibrations. The study of Ayurveda, combined with a knowledge of *swar* yoga[*]—the science of breath—provides a complete road map for the practitioner.

To acquire knowledge of anatomy and physiology, the practitioner may chose to study textbooks and take formal classes, as well as participate in martial arts classes and engage in weight lifting and bodybuilding. To acquire an understanding of the natural shape of the spine, the practitioner should study happy and healthy children, three to eight years of age. Observation is key to the study of the human physique. It is critical to have a keen eye and also to study one's own body.

Strokes

The four types of strokes that should be used in Ayurvedic massage are tapping, kneading, rubbing, and squeezing. The practitioner should start by tapping the area to be massaged, and then kneading the same area. Then a few drops of oil should be vigorously rubbed between the palms to increase the circulation and warmth of the practitioner's hands. This warmth will stimulate the lymph nodes and the flow of lymph in the recipient's body. Then the oil should be rubbed on the body. Each time physical contact is broken, the practitioner should vigorously clap his or her hands. This serves to give the recipient some breathing time and to revitalize the practitioner's energy. Once a body part has been thoroughly rubbed, the practitioner ends with a crisscross movement, squeezing the muscles with both hands.

---

* See *Breath, Mind, and Consciousness* by Harish Johari (Rochester, Vermont: Destiny Books, 1989) for more information on swar yoga.

TAPPING

Tapping awakens the body. It increases blood circulation and excites the capillaries under the skin, making the muscles strong. It also serves to activate the nervous system. Tapping alerts the body's natural defenses that the massage has begun. Tapping should be done with cupped palms. One minute of tapping equalizes the temperature between the hands of the practitioner and the area of the body being massaged.

KNEADING

While tapping increases the flow of life force (prana) into a particular area, kneading relaxes and removes the stress that has accumulated in the muscles, joints, and ligaments during the activities of daily life. Muscles should be kneaded like a baker kneads dough and works with its texture. As muscles loosen and the toughness caused by stress dissolves, the muscles will begin to feel like well-kneaded dough. Kneading creates activity inside the cell walls, increasing the circulation of the life-giving chemicals that help develop and rejuvenate the body. After kneading the practitioner should grasp the muscle and shake it a bit to see if the loosening process has made it smooth. If the musculature does not become relaxed and loose enough, the nutritional oil will not be properly absorbed and assimilated. Once the muscles are sufficiently soft, the next step—rubbing—can begin.

RUBBING

Dry rubbing provides exercise for the skin: it excites the circulation of blood and lymph and increases heat in the area being massaged. This stimulation permits nutrients present in the ciculatory system to reach the joints, and thus strengthens the bones. Dry rubbing also alleviates stiff muscles and removes fatigue. While rubbing the skin dry with a rough towel after a bath does provide benefits, it can also disturb the body gases by means of increasing vayu, the wind element. For this reason, a rough towel should only be used after a bath and only under therapeutic advice.

Some Hindu and Jain sadhus rub ashes on their bodies, which creates a kind of immunity in them to the sense of touch. By desensitizing their skin—the organ that receives the sense of touch—they are protected from seasonal changes. The ashes become their clothes. This practice, however, is only for initiates in the Hindu or Jain orders. Anyone else attempting this would develop dry skin that could peel or become sore.

Oil rubbing, with an oil suitable for the season and the aggravated dosha, is generally recommended by Ayurveda. If pain, swelling, or a rash occurs, then an oil suitable for these conditions should be used.

Properly used, oil can be very beneficial. In addition to not exciting the vayu element and thus disturbing body gases, it lubricates the fingers, facilitates the rubbing, and distributes the body temperature evenly. If the oil is fragrant, it also generates a pleasant aroma and so creates a pleasant environment for the massage. (For oils with no fragrance, a few drops of an organic essential oil may be added).

Rubbing the top, sides, and bottom of a joint helps its articulation and movement because the lymph nodes, which are situated around the joints to keep them lubricated and protected from friction, are stimulated and release lymphatic fluid (see page 22). Depending on how it is done, rubbing serves different purposes. Gentle rubbing helps the recipient to relax, while hard rubbing produces the benefits of exercise. The practitioner should start rubbing gently, applying the oil to the area that is to be massaged. After the oil has been applied, the rubbing can be done harder to create heat and allow the oil be absorbed by the body. The speed at which the practitioner works should complement the touch: when the massage is gentle, the cadence should be slow; when it become more rigorous, the speed should increase somewhat. After the rubbing, the practitioner should make circular movements on the marmas (pressure points) as described in the chapters that follow.

SQUEEZING

The fourth and final massage technique, squeezing, is done only to the limbs, fingers, and toes. After the oil used during rubbing has been absorbed,* squeeze the body part by making a crisscross movement with both hands. Squeezing should start at the thighs and move downward to the tips of the toes, and then begin again at the armpit and end at the fingertips. Squeezing the fingers and toes is like milking a cow, except that the squeezing movement runs crisscross while the milking movement is straight downward. By gently twisting the bones of the toes and fingers at the joint to either side, the secretion of growth hormones will be stimulated.

Squeezing influences the fine network of nerves and blood capillaries lying underneath the skin and forces the flow of nutrient material toward the extremities. Done with bearable pressure, this movement balances the pressure of blood and other fluids inside the cell walls. By creating an even distribution of energy, squeezing helps to balance the musculature. Through squeezing, tension and pain in the arms and legs are released through the fingers and toes.

After the limbs have all been squeezed and the recipient is relaxing, the practitioner should apply a drop of oil to each of the recipient's fingertips. Oil is then carefully placed around the tip of each toenail, filling the area between the flesh and the nail itself. Repeat until all toenails have been oiled. This removes

---

* When the oil has been absorbed, the thin film becomes invisible and oil does not wipe off on a clean cloth.

dryness and makes the pads of the toes, which become hard and cracked, smooth again. It also smoothes and strengthens the nails.

DIRECTION OF MASSAGE

The body can be grouped into four sections: From the base of the spine to the base of the skull (back of torso and head); from the collarbone to the fingertips (front and back of arms and hands); from the pelvis to the toes (front and back of pelvis, legs, and feet); and the head and ears.

Base of the Spine to Base of the Skull

This region of the body is the first to develop as a unit in utero. After fertilization of the ovum, the head is the first body part to develop, followed by the torso. In this region the energy moves in two directions: up the back and down the front. For this reason, massage on the back should begin at the base of the spine and move upward along both sides of the vertebral column simultaneously, to the base of the skull.

If the massage is given in reverse order, from the neck toward the pelvis, energy is drawn downward with the hands and sensual games can begin. With the upward flow of energy, thoughts are integrated and mental problems solved. Also, while massaging the back properly, each vertebra gets properly aligned.

The Collarbone to the Fingertips

This region includes the upper arms, elbows, forearms, wrists, palms, and fingers. Energy is drawn into the body through these parts. The hands are used to draw in, pull, express emotions, and protect oneself. Hands thus serve as a vehicle of both prana and the mind. In dance, they express emotions through mudras (hand postures); in worship they serve as connectors, raising the energy level and helping channel psychic currents. By engaging the fingers, the mind can become one-pointed and centered. Fingers connect the mind with the world outside—they express mental states and thoughts.

The flow of energy travels from the collarbone towards the fingertips, from the inside of the arm to the outside. For this reason, massage is done downward from the collarbone to the fingertips.

Pelvis to Toes

In this region, energy circulates in a downward direction. The feet are in constant contact with the earth and its gravitational force. In India, people touch the feet of elders to obtain their blessings and receive the loving energy transmitted through their feet. Scriptural verses praise the lotus feet of the guru; meditation on the guru's feet is said to bring peace and destroy all sin. *Shaktipat mahayoga*, a yogic path that believes in the transference of energy, states that the feet of the guru are worshiped because it is through them that the guru transfers his or her energy to the disciple. This energy helps open the knots *(grantis)* that impede the flow of energy to higher psychic centers (chakras), freeing energy for higher states of consciousness. It is said that Ramakrishna Paramahamsa transferred his energy into his disciple Narendra (later known as Vivekananda) by kicking him at the base of his spine.

Thus, in keeping with the direction in which energy circulates in the body, massage of this region is done from the pelvis toward the toes. If the massage is done in reverse order, the muscles of the legs will suffer ill effects and the hair follicles will be irritated.

The Head and Ears

Head massage starts with measuring eight fingerwidths from the eyebrows to the top of the cranium. Oil is poured on the point of the fontanel (the soft spot). The oil is then spread sideways. Then oil is poured on the place where the hairs turn in a cowlick. Again the oil is spread with both hands on both sides of the head. Finally, oil is poured on the junction of the neck and the skull and is then spread on the area of the neck and back of the skull.

SEQUENCE OF MASSAGE

In Ayurveda, massage starts with the lower half of the body to relax the entire being. Working on the feet, which have many reflex points corresponding to the rest of the body, is done at the beginning to prepare the body for the torso massage. This is followed by work on the upper back and arms. Then the upper torso is done, followed by the arms. The head, which is massaged last, is massaged while the recipient is in a seated position. (Because circulation is not normal when we recline, this position is not suitable for working on the head and face.) This particular sequence systematically energizes and relaxes, allowing the effects of the massage to accrue.

To receive the maximum benefit from an Ayurvedic massage, the following sequence should be followed:

BACK OF BODY

1. Pelvis to toes (left and right sides), moving downward

2. Spine—tailbone to neck—moving upward

3. Shoulder blades to fingers, moving downward (left and right sides)

FRONT OF BODY

1. Pelvis to toes (left and right sides), moving downward

2. Navel to chest, moving upward

3. Collarbone to fingers, moving downward (left and right sides)

SEATED POSITION

1. Inside of upper arm to fingertips (left and right sides)

2. Neck, skull, and face, massaging from back to front

It is important to understand the bipolar nature of the limbs. The outside of a limb, which is farther from the spine, is rough and can bear more temperature and pressure changes than the inside. The outside aspect is considered male, while the inside is considered female. While the outside is less sensitive and less ticklish, it accumulates more fatigue and holds more tension and therefore should be massaged first.

The massage recipient needs to wear a minimal amount of clothing. Before beginning, he or she should be asked to assume the corpse posture for a few minutes to loosen the body. To assume this posture, known as shavasana in the yogic scriptures, give the recipient the following instructions.

> Lie flat on your back, with your feet shoulder-width apart and arms resting comfortably by your side, palms up. With eyes closed, let your mind become calm and passive. Direct your attention to your toes and feet and release any tension that may exist there. Concentrate on the knees, thighs, abdomen, chest, and head in the same way, allowing them to become relaxed and open. After a few minutes of total relaxation, check the entire body again to be sure no tensions are present. Then concentrate on the third eye—the region between the eyebrows—and remain in the corpse pose for a few minutes more. Now you can stand and take a breath, slowly stretching your arms up along your sides while inhaling. Exhale and release the arms back to gravity. Repeat this stretch a few times, with the rhythm of the breath.

As the recipient does this slow stretch, the practitioner can note whether the body is erect or tilted. Often people tilt to one side or the other while believing they are standing straight. If the person cannot, upon request, align the shoulders, then additional time should be spent on the higher shoulder during the massage. The recipient should also be advised to keep an awareness of standing erect in general, which will help mental balance as well. If the person cannot

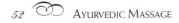

stand erect at will, he or she should be asked to become aware of which nostril is dominant over the course of the next thirty days. This will reveal which hemisphere of the brain is dominant (the left hemisphere dominates the right side of the body and vice versa). Then the recipient should be advised to change the nostril frequently, so as to reestablish a hemispheric balance.[*]

POST-MASSAGE

Once the massage is complete, the recipient should resume the corpse pose.[†] The practitioner should cover the recipient with a clean sheet, and then also assume the corpse pose in a nearby comfortable place (the floor will do). In this way both participants can relax and reestablish their normal breathing patterns. The rhythm of the breath often increases with massage.

---

[*] To change the dominant nostril, lie down on the side of the operating nostril and place a small cushion under the rib cage to provide pressure to the lung on that side.

[†] If the massage is being done for health and beauty, the recipient should stand up and walk slowly for a few minutes before assuming the corpse posture.

Chapter Five

Full-Body Massage

The full-body massage described in this chapter focuses on the marmas, which is how the pressure points are known in Ayurveda. The names of the marmas and their location on the body are listed on pages 41–43; for quick reference, the marmas are listed in alphabetical order in the Appendix.

While learning this massage practice, the reader should continually refer to the Marma Charts in the Appendix (pages 136–41) in order to determine the exact location of each marma. You may want to photocopy the charts and the alphabetical list, keeping them alongside the book for easy reference as you practice.

GENERAL GUIDELINES FOR AYURVEDIC MASSAGE

1. The fingerwidths, which are used as units of measure in the instructions that follow, refer to the fingerwidth *of the recipient*. They can be approximated.

2. Clap your hands each time you remove them from the recipient's body. This practice is traditionally used in Indian massage to relax and recharge the hands of the practitioner.

3. When massaging marmas, make small concentric circles with your fingertips. Move clockwise with your right hand and counterclockwise with your left hand.

4. Certain marmas are located in both the arms and legs, and so have the same names.

5. Marmas can receive pressure from two directions. When a marma can be rubbed from front and back, it is referred to as having *anterior* and *posterior* aspects, as with the janu marma on the knee. When a marma can be rubbed from both sides, it is referred to as having *lateral* and *medial* aspects, as with the gulpha marma on the ankle.

6. Marmas can be intentionally "blocked." This is done by pressing or holding the marma point with the thumb in order to briefly allow the energy or circulating fluids to flow around the marma.

PREPARATION

Place a thin futon covered with a soft straw mat on the floor. (The straw mat saves the futon from getting stained by oil.) You may dress in loose comfortable clothing. Ask the recipient to remove all but his or her underwear. It is advised that men and women massage only people of their own gender, to prevent being distracted by sexual energy.

Ask the recipient to lie in a supine position on the mat in the shavasana pose (see page 51) and relax. Pull each ankle gently to stretch the legs and realign the muscles and joints. Then ask the recipient to turn over, with arms resting in a comfortable position. Squat, with your legs spread over the thighs of the recipient, or kneel or sit to the side to execute the massage.

Shake your hands until a tingling sensation is felt in the fingertips. Then rotate your wrists alternately to the left and right, or move your hands rhythmically, as if you were making mudras in an Indian dance. Shake your wrists once again a little faster. When the tingling sensation is felt this time, the fingers are charged with fresh energy. Rub your palms together to generate a bit more warmth, and then begin the massage.

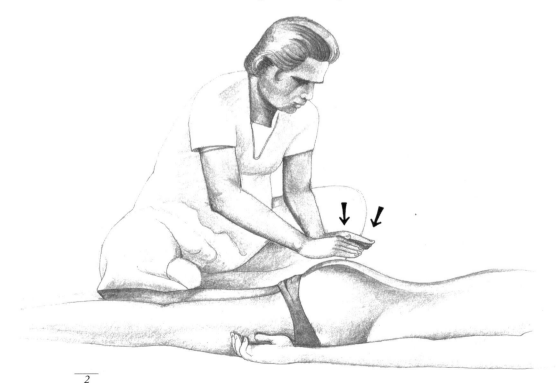

LOWER BACK OF THE BODY

Massage of the Buttocks and Hips

Rounding your palms to create a cuplike shape, start tapping the hips and base of the spine with both hands (fig. 2). Tapping enhances circulation and signals the cells that the massage is starting. After one minute, start kneading the buttocks with both hands, applying gentle pressure (fig. 3). Then press the buttocks in a pinching fashion with thumbs and fingertips, or palms and fingertips, to excite the fine capillaries of the vascular system (fig. 4). This pressing movement briefly interrupts the blood flow. Once pressure is removed, the blood rushes forth with greater intensity, activating the circulatory system and enhancing toxin release.

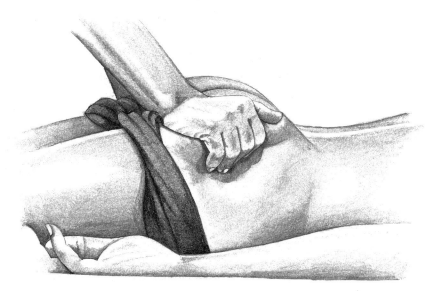

3

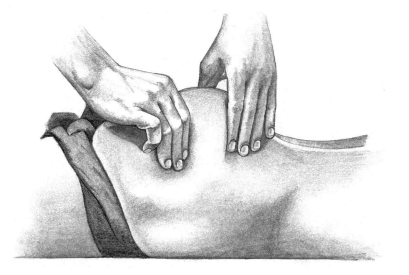

4

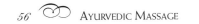

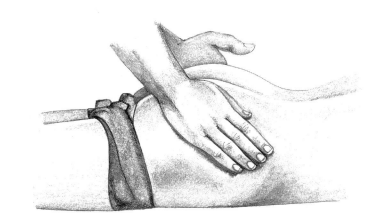

5

After pressing, place your hands on either side of the recipient's hips and shake the buttock muscles back and forth like gelatin, to loosen and soften the tissue (fig. 5). Apply oil to your hands and place your thumbs on either side of the tailbone, about 1 inch above the tip. The fingers of each of your hands will

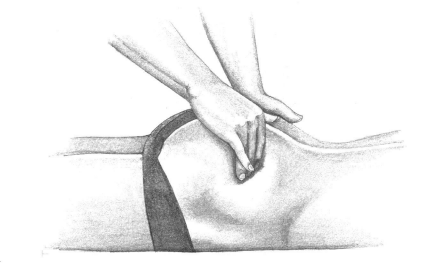

6

naturally be resting above the nitamba marmas (fig. 6). Press both your hands on these marmas, making small concentric circles. Release your thumbs and rub the marmas with oil, gradually increasing the size of the circles until you encompass the full surface of the buttock area (fig. 7). Continue rubbing with your palms until the oil is completely spread and absorbed. Apply more oil if needed to make the muscles smooth to the touch and shiny. Remove your thumbs

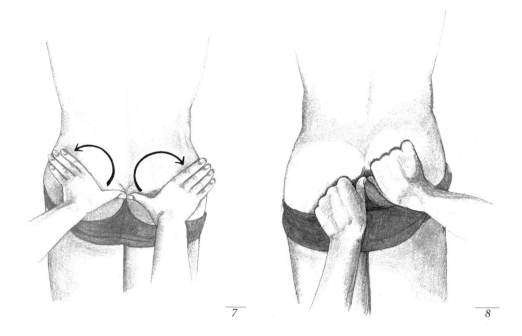

7

8

from the sacrum area and gradually reduce the size of the concentric circles. End massage of the hips with your fingertips on the nitamba marmas. Before leaving the area, press gently for a moment on the guda marma, located on the tip of the tailbone (fig. 8).

Massage of the Upper Leg

Begin by tapping the tops and sides of both thighs. To loosen the muscles, place your hands on either side of one thigh and shake back and forth. Then knead the thigh muscles using bearable pressure, alternating hands as you knead (fig. 9). Once the muscles have relaxed, pour a little oil on your hands and apply to the top and sides of the thigh. Locate two marmas with your thumbs: the posterior

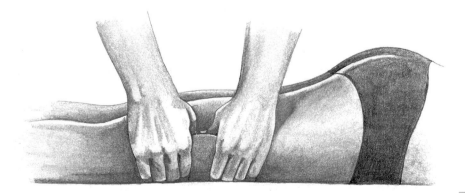

9

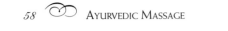

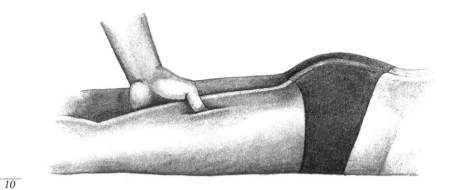

10

urvi marma, just above the midpoint of the thigh (fig. 10), and the posterior ani, three fingerwidths above janu (fig. 11). Massage each point using small concentric circles. Because marmas are situated at the juncture of muscles, bones, ligaments, arteries, and nerves, a pulsation can be felt on these spots.

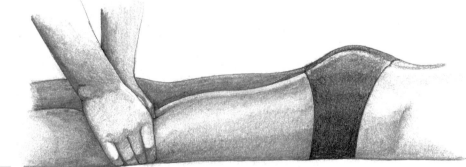

11

Once the marmas are rubbed, the muscles should also be massaged. Place your thumbs in the center of the thigh near the gluteal fold, with palms resting on either side. Move down the thigh, applying pressure primarily on the outside of the thigh. (The inner thigh will be massaged properly later.) When you reach the knee, lighten your touch and circle back toward the starting point. The oil should be completely absorbed and the massaged area should be soft, smooth in texture, and warm to the touch. The color of the skin should be pink compared to the area that has not been massaged.

Again, return your thumbs to the center of the thigh under the gluteal fold, resting your inside hand near the inguinal lymph nodes. Squeeze the upper leg, crisscrossing your hands until you reach the knee (fig. 12). Move both hands toward and then away from each other. Repeat this squeezing motion three times, massaging from the upper thigh to the knee.

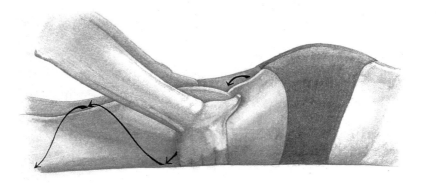

12

Behind the knee is a fine network of lymph nodes and a marma known as posterior janu. This point, located in the middle of the knee, should pulsate beneath your thumb. Make a circular movement with three fingers on this point (fig. 13). Gently rub the entire area behind the knee with oiled fingertips (fig. 14) to stimulate the lymph nodes.

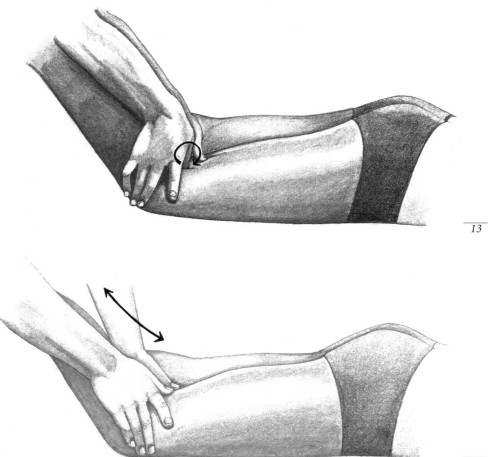

13

14

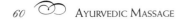

Massage of the Lower Leg

From a kneeling position, place the front of the recipient's foot on your thigh. After tapping the calf vigorously from knee to ankle, hold both sides of the calf and shake the muscles back and forth (fig. 15). Since the calves carry the weight of the entire upper body, they accumulate stress and become hard and sore. Relaxing these muscles and restoring their flexibility is essential.

On the midline of the calf muscle, six fingerwidths down from the knee crease, is the indravasti marma. Apply gentle pressure on this point with your thumb and then rub it with oil. Holding the front of the ankle up with one hand, use the other hand to apply bearable pressure to the outside of the calf, rubbing oil well into the muscle (fig. 16). For this move, the thumb remains on the midline of the calf muscle. When the hand reaches the ankle, make a circular pass upward without pressure, returning to the starting point. Repeat several times, until the calf muscle is soft and relaxed and the oil has been absorbed. Then hold the ankle with your other hand and rub the inside of the calf muscle in the same way.

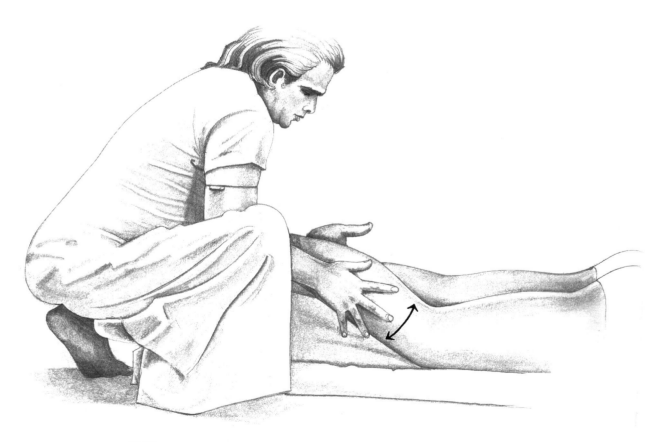

15

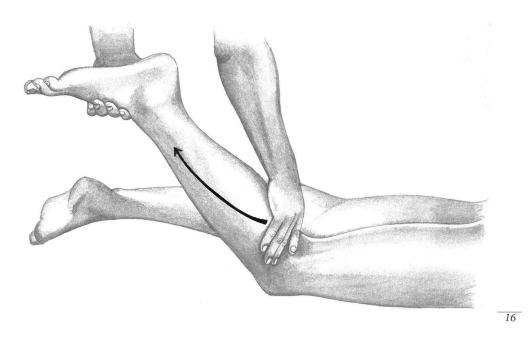

16

Hold the top of the foot with one hand and apply oil on ankle area with the other. The gulpha marma is located on the ankle bone. Rub the medial and lateral aspects of the gulpha point gently with oil (fig. 17).

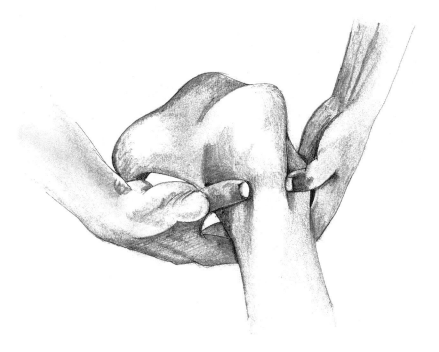

17

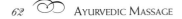

Massage of the Feet (Soles Only)

The feet are said to contain reflex points to all organs and parts of the body. In classical drawings of the feet, these energies are represented by symbols (fig. 18). According to the Indian scriptures, diseases do not go near one who massages his legs and feet from knee to toes before sleeping, just as snakes do not approach eagles. A physician who studied these points while he was visiting India determined the connection of these points with internal organs and thus began foot reflexology as it is known in the West. If the soles of the feet are regularly pressed and rubbed with oil or beeswax cream,* a person will remain relaxed and healthy.

A simple oil massage of the feet prevents cracking and peeling of the skin due to cold weather. It eliminates or reduces infections caused by fungus and bacteria; it also soothes an agitated mind.

Foot massage is important in part because the feet contain so many joints, or sandhis. Fifteen sandhis can be found in each foot: two in the big toe, three in each remaining toe, and one in the ankle. (The leg proper contains two sandhis: the knee joint and the hip joint.) Lymph nodes exist within each joint. Flexibility in these joints is essential.

To work on the soles of the feet, apply oil to your palms. While holding the front of the foot, rub and press the sole, moving forward and back (fig. 19). No tapping or kneading is required on this area. End each downward stroke with a

18

A traditional rendering of Vishnu Charan, the feet of Lord Vishnu.

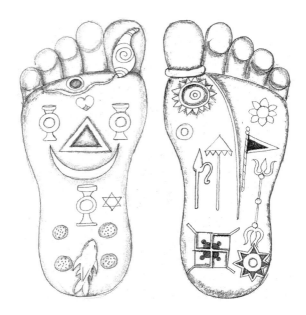

---

* Beeswax cream does not stain fabrics. For a recipe on how to make it at home, see page 134. Beeswax cream helps keep the skin moist, prevents skin diseases, and strengthens the nerves. Only a small amount is needed to cover the feet or face.

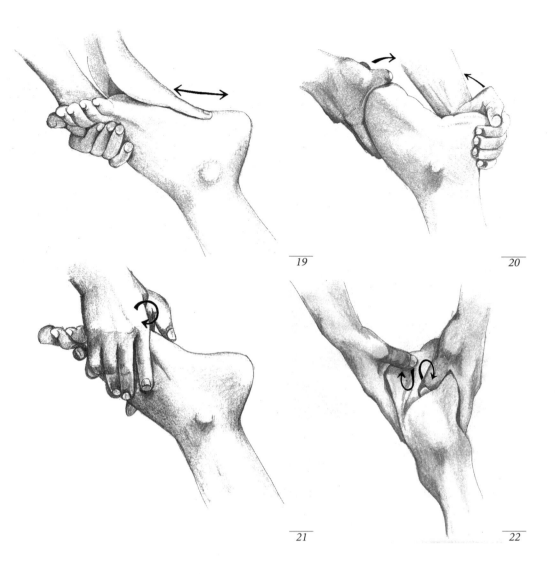

19

20

21

22

stretch, gently pressing into the arch of the foot by drawing the heel and toes toward each other (fig. 20). Four marmas are situated on the sole of each foot: kurchshira, talhridaya, kuruchcha, and kshipra. Rub these marmas, using gentle pressure (figs. 21 and 22).

The massage of the lower leg and foot ends with a squeezing of the leg three times, from knee to toes. Overlap the hands and use a crisscross motion, much like the squeezing of the thigh shown in figure 12. The overall leg massage culminates with a single squeeze of the entire leg, from the top of the thigh to the toes.

Repeat the leg massage on the opposite leg, starting with the thigh (see page 57). Once both legs have been massaged, ask the recipient to turn over, keeping the legs relaxed and slightly separated.

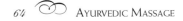

LOWER FRONT OF THE BODY

Massage of the Upper Leg

Start the massage on the side of the body that corresponds to the operating nostril (see page 52). Kneel over the recipient's thigh, or sit to the side if that is more comfortable.

Gently tap the outside of the thigh, then the inside. Place the thigh between your palms and shake the muscles back and forth like gelatin (fig. 23). Apply oil to your hands and knead the outer thigh muscles a few minutes. The outside is

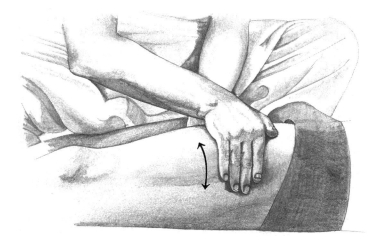

23

the male or electrical side of the body; it accumulates more tension than the inside. Massaging this area first removes muscular tension and stress. The inside is the female or magnetic side, which contains many lymph nodes.

Using the middle fingers, make small circular strokes on the two marmas located near the thigh/torso juncture: lohitaksha, situated in the middle of the thigh, and vitapam, found at the beginning of the testicles in men and about four fingerwidths above the genital organ in women (fig. 24). Try to feel the pulsation before applying pressure to the marma.

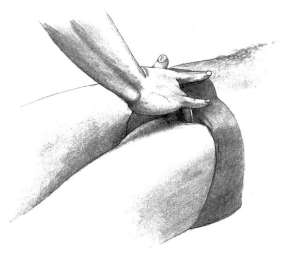

24

Rub and press the muscles on the outer thigh with your palms, making several large oval movements from hip joint to knee. Every now and then hold a muscle band between your thumbs and fingers and press (fig. 25). Each time you remove your hands from the body, clap them and shake them out to avoid storing tension in your fingers and wrists. Continue working on the outer thigh until the oil has been absorbed; the muscles should become warm, smooth, and pliable.

Just above and slightly lateral to the kneecap is the ani marma. Massage it in small circular movements, as you have the other marmas.

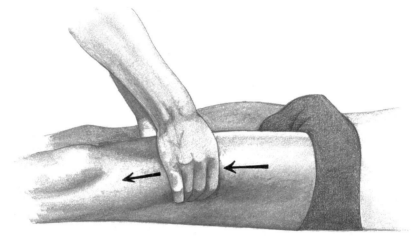

25

To massage the inner thigh, begin by gently tapping the inside of the thigh. Place hands on either side of the thigh. With one hand resting on the outer thigh, shake the inner thigh muscles with fingers of your other hand (see fig. 23). Oil your hands and knead the muscles of the inner thigh for a few minutes. Rub and press simultaneously with your fingers and palms. (Pressing here is a pinching of the muscles between your thumb and fingers.) In the middle of the inner thigh is a marma known as the anterior urvi (fig. 26). Massage it in small circular movements, as you have the other marmas.

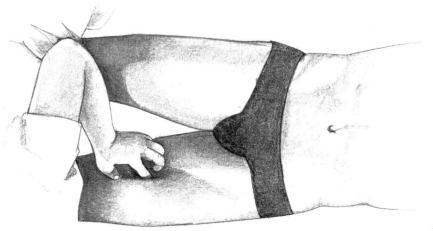

26

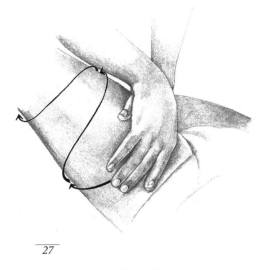

27

After massaging the outer and inner thigh, squeeze the entire upper leg. To do this, ask the recipient to bend his knee. Place your thumbs near the groin, fingers resting on either side of the thigh (fig. 27). Start by moving your hands toward each other, applying bearable pressure. When your hands cross at the front of the thigh, move them apart again. Your hands move downward with each crisscrossing, until they reach the knee. Repeat this squeezing of the upper leg three times.

Massage of the Knee

Although the area being covered is small, massage of the knee is somewhat complicated. Kneeling in front of the leg to be worked on, place one hand behind the calf and rest the recipient's foot against your thigh. While holding the calf muscle with one hand, rotate the kneecap gently with your other hand in a clockwise direction (fig. 28).

Two marmas, ani and janu, can be found near the knee. The anterior ani is located just above and lateral to the kneecap and the posterior janu is located behind the knee in the center of the knee crease.

With one hand, place your thumb on the anterior ani and your middle finger on the posterior janu. Place the thumb of your opposite hand on the anterior janu, located on the inner knee just below the kneecap, and the middle finger on the posterior janu. In the final position, your two middle fingers are on same

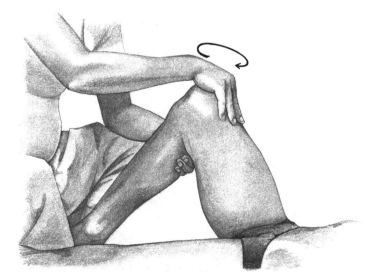

28

point behind the knee (the posterior janu) and your thumbs rest diagonally across the knee, one on the anterior ani marma and the other on the anterior janu marma (fig. 29). Massage these three points simultaneously, moving clockwise with the right hand and counterclockwise with the left.

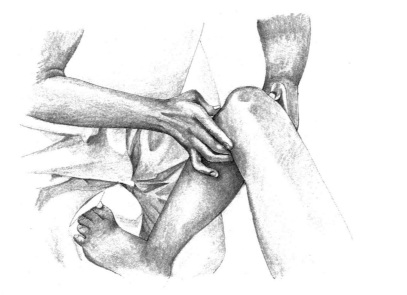

29

While continuing to hold these marma points, check that the recipient's foot rests securely against your thigh and does not slide down. Then grip the top of the calf with the last three fingers of both hands, gently massaging the entire janu area behind the knee with downward strokes (fig. 30). This will stimulate the many lymph nodes located behind the knee.

To end the knee massage, repeat the position shown in figure 29, and rub the two marmas on the front of the knee again with your thumbs.

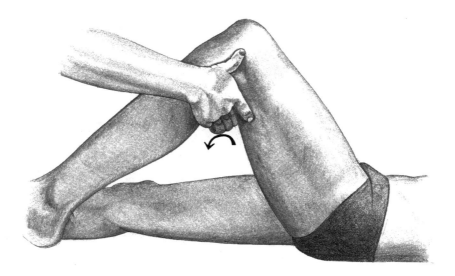

30

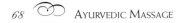

Massage of the Calf

Although the calves were done earlier in this massage sequence, they normally hold a lot of stress and can only benefit by the repetition.

Keep the leg in a bent position, with the sole of the foot resting against your thigh. Begin by tapping the calf muscle from top to bottom a few times. Then, holding the calf between your palms, shake it back and forth like gelatin until it becomes loose and soft. Follow this by kneading the calf muscles with your palms and fingers, from knee to ankle (fig. 31). Once the kneading is complete, apply oil to your hands and rub the calf with cup-shaped palms. The pressure here can be a little harder than that used on the thighs. Make repetitive, sweeping strokes with your cupped palms, moving from knee to ankle (fig. 32). These strokes will excite the capillaries and nerves. Gradually increase your speed and strength until a clapping sound is produced when your cupped palms meet the calf muscles.

Locate the indravasti marma, situated in the middle of the gastrocnemius muscle, and gently rub (fig. 33). Also press the pressure points (these are not marmas) that register most of the tension, located on either side of the calf muscle.

Complete the massage of the lower leg with a squeezing stroke. Cross your thumbs just below the kneecap, with fingers resting on either side of the calf. Move your hands in a crisscross movement, squeezing the lower leg from knee to ankle (fig. 34). Repeat three times.

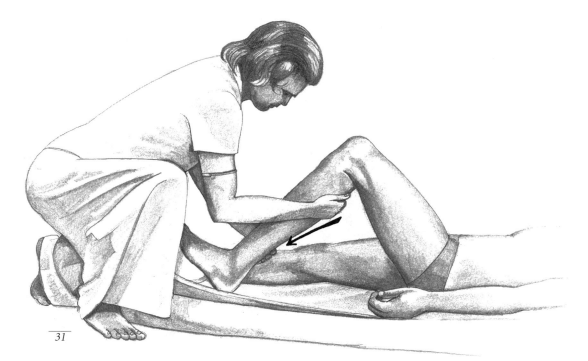

31

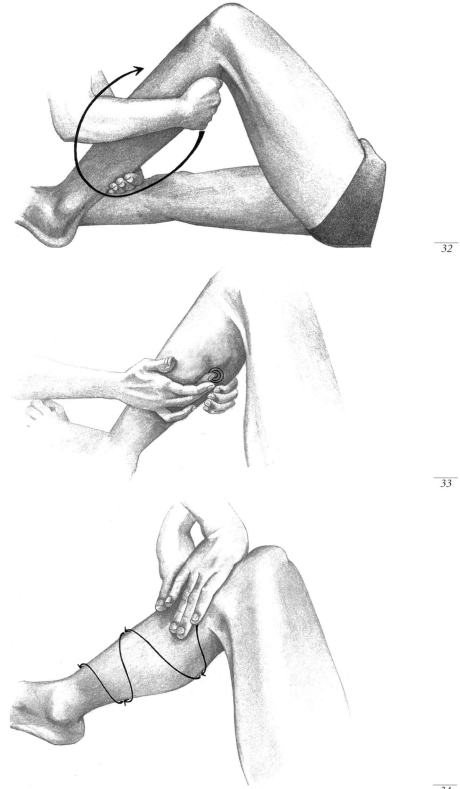

32

33

34

Massage of the Foot

Since the ankle is a comparatively narrow area, only your fingers and thumbs need to be used. Tapping, kneading, and shaking are not necessary because there are so few muscles. While holding the calf with one hand, dip the fingertips of your opposite hand in oil; using your thumb, index and middle fingers, rub downward, creating a chain of small circles (fig. 35). Then rub all around the ankle bone.

Locate the kurchshira and gulpha marmas at the heel and the outer ankle joint respectively (fig. 36), and rub them in a circular fashion as you have the other marmas. Applying simultaneous pressure to the lateral and medial aspects of the gulpha marma can bring relief to the condition of sciatica.

With one hand supporting the foot above the heel, wrap your other hand around the toes. First gently stretch and bend the foot in all directions to loosen it. Then, still supporting the heel, grasp the toes and rotate the top of the foot (fig. 37). (The left foot rotates clockwise and right foot rotates counterclockwise.)

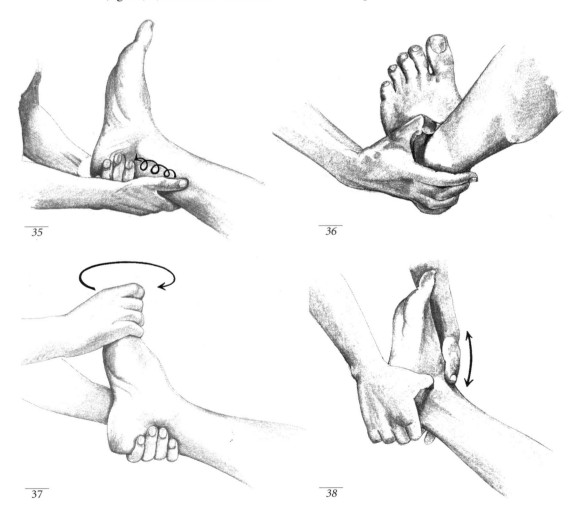

35

36

37

38

When the foot is relaxed, block the medial gulpha marma (inner heel) with your thumb while pressing on the lateral kurchshira marma with your middle finger (fig. 38). Dip the fingers of your opposite hand in oil and press firmly along the outer edge of the foot toward the toes. Repeat these steps, except this time block the medial kurchshira marma with your thumb while pressing on the lateral gulpha marma with your middle finger. Again, with the oiled fingers of your other hand press along the lateral edge of the foot toward the toes.

Once both marmas have been blocked medially, the process is reversed and they are blocked laterally. Block the lateral gulpha marma (outer heel) with your thumb while pressing on the medial kurchshira marma with your middle finger. Dip the fingers of your opposite hand in oil and press firmly along the medial edge of the foot, toward the toenails. Repeat these steps, except this time block lateral kurchshira marma with your thumb while pressing on the medial gulpha marma with your middle finger. Again, with the oiled fingers of your opposite hand, press along the medial edge of the foot toward the toes.

To begin working on the toes, block the lateral kurchshira marma with the thumb of your opposite hand. Continue to block this marma as you work with the big toe and the second toe. Place your thumb between the joints of the big toe and second toe, and rub in a clockwise direction (fig. 39). Press and rub the first joint of the second toe from both sides (fig. 40). (The location of this joint is shown as I in figure 40.) Then hold the joint with thumb and forefinger and gently twist. Twist the remaining two joints, moving toward the tip of the toe. (The locations of these joints are shown as II and III in figure 40.) Now release the lateral kurchshira and block the medial kurchshira as you do gentle joint twists on the remaining three toes. Release the marma and, holding the second

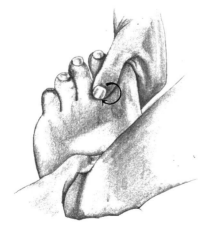

39

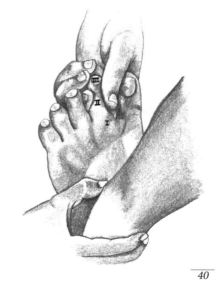

40

toe between your thumb and forefinger, pull it toward you (fig. 41). Allow the toe to crack as it lengthens, and press it tightly for a moment before releasing. Repeat this treatment on the three remaining toes.

The big toe has only two joints. To massage these joints, use the hand that was blocking the marmas as support under the outer edge of foot. Placing the thumb and index finger of your free hand on either side of the first joint, press and twist. Repeat on the second joint. Apply pressure on the second joint and pull the big toe, allowing it to crack. Try again to pull any toes that did not crack the first time. Finally, hold all toes firmly in your grip while simultaneously pressing and lengthening them.

When you have finished, pour a drop of oil on each toenail (fig. 42). This stops hardening and cracking of the nails and makes them shiny and beautiful.

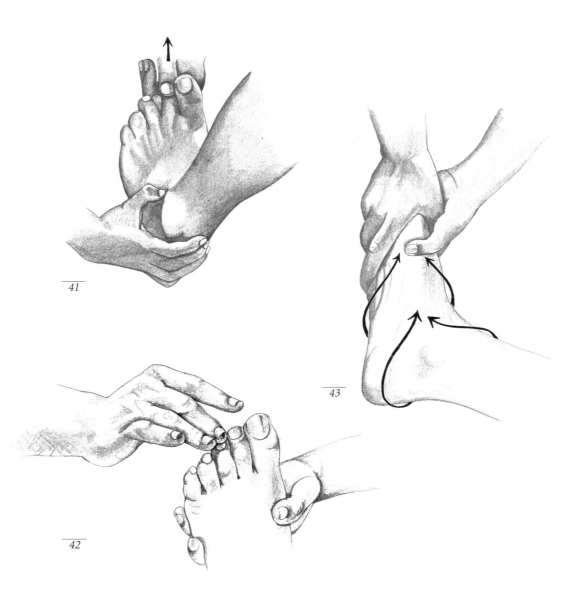

41

43

42

End massage of the leg by clapping your hands to recharge them. Return to the torso/thigh juncture and squeeze the entire leg, using a crisscross movement, until you reach the toes (figs. 27, 34, and 43). Repeat this squeezing of the leg three times.

Return to the section entitled Massage of the Upper Leg (page 57) and repeat all the steps on the opposite leg. When both legs have been completed, continue with massage of the back as described below.

ABOUT THE BACK

On either side of the spinal column lie the sympathetic ganglia, major relay stations for nerve impulses of the sympathetic nervous system. Massage of this area helps to put the spine in proper alignment and strengthens the nervous system. It also enhances circulation of cerebrospinal fluid and increases the discharge of neurons. While the leg massage works mostly on the lymphatic system, massage of the spine is related to the autonomic (sympathetic and parasympathetic) nervous system.

According to the ancient system of Tantra, the human organism has seven subtle centers of consciousness, or chakras, five of which are specified along the spinal column. These five chakras work with the basic elements—Earth, Water, Fire, Air, and Akash—which are the building blocks of the external world of names and forms. The entire human organism is an interplay of these five elements. While chakras cannot be massaged directly because they form part of the subtle (nonphysical) body, they are linked to the organs of the physical body (through the nervous system and the endocrine glands), and are thus able to be affected by massage.

The spine houses a network of subtle nerves called nadis that connect to the visceral organs and sense organs of these psychic centers.

1. The base of the spine aligns with the first chakra

2. The lowest aspect of the iliac crest (the ASIS) aligns with the second chakra

3. The bottom of the rib cage aligns with the third chakra

4. The bottom of the shoulder blades aligns with the fourth chakra

5. The bottom of the collarbone aligns with the fifth chakra

To stimulate the five psychic centers described above, have the recipient turn over and lie in a prone position, arms folded under the forehead. Place your knees on either side of the recipient's thighs. This will provide you access to the back of the body from the tailbone to the cerebellum. Move your fingers in a straight line from point to point along the spine. Rub each one with your thumb in a circular movement, moving up from the tailbone.

MASSAGE OF THE BACK

Now we will continue with the remainder of the back massage. Ask the recipient to breathe deeply and slowly, holding the air in as long as is comfortable. The two areas in the back that are often stressed and in need of attention are the waist and the shoulder area. During the back massage, your thumbs will work on either side of the spinal column while your palms and fingers will work on the rest of the back area (fig. 44). Movements are always made toward the head. Extra kneading and pressing should be done on areas that are especially painful; generally, this can be continued until the pain dissipates. Remember to clap your hands each time you remove them from the recipient's body in order to recharge them.

Start the back massage by tapping the tailbone area. Fix your thumbs on the tip of the tailbone. Rub and press in the direction of the sacrum. At the waist region begin tapping with cupped hands again (fig. 45). Grasping the muscles at the lower waist, shake them and then knead them (fig. 46), first on one side and then the other.

Apply oil to your hands and spread it with a circular motion on both sides of the waist simultaneously, using bearable pressure (fig. 47). Find the kukundaraya marmas, located on either sacroiliac joint six fingerwidths up from the tip of the coccyx. Hold the kukundaraya marmas with your thumbs as you massage the katika tarunam marmas on the pelvic crest; release your thumbs and rub the parshva sandhi marmas with your middle fingers (fig. 48). The parshva sandhi marmas sit four fingerwidths above the katika tarunam marmas.

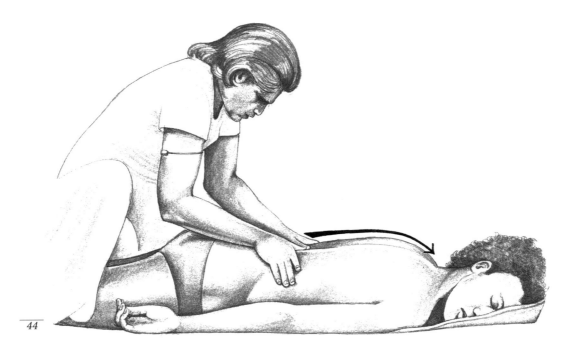

44

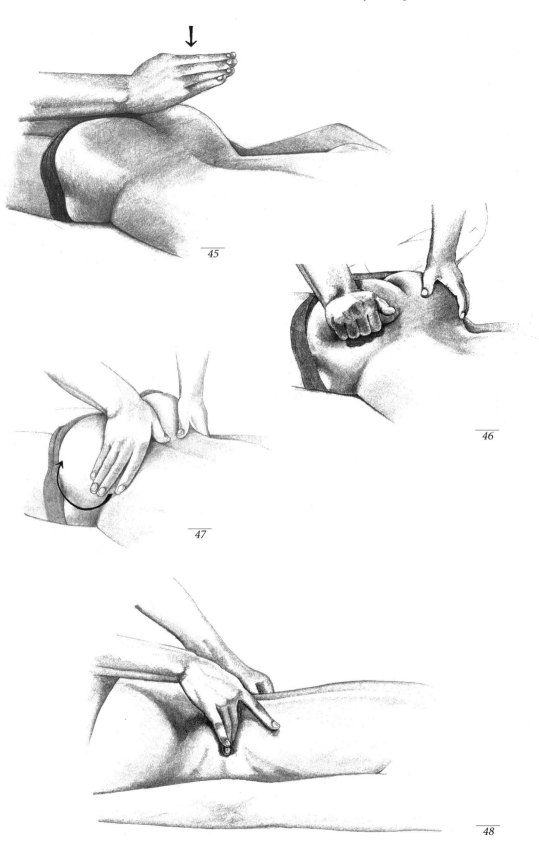

45

46

47

48

Move up the spine to the vrihati marmas located on either side of the 10th thoracic vertebra. Rub this marma, then move upward and rub in a circular direction toward the outside of each shoulder blade (fig. 49). Finish the shoulder massage with a long kneading (fig. 50).

Locate the six marmas in the neck region—the two krikatikas and the four siramatrikas. Begin by rubbing the two krikatikas marmas with your thumbs. These marmas are located where the spine joins the skull. Then rub the four posterior siramatrika marmas, located on either side of the neck. After gently rubbing these marmas, you and the recipient should relax for a short while. (As these marmas are easier to view in an illustration in which the recipient is in a seated position, please see figures 85 and 86 for the marma locations.)

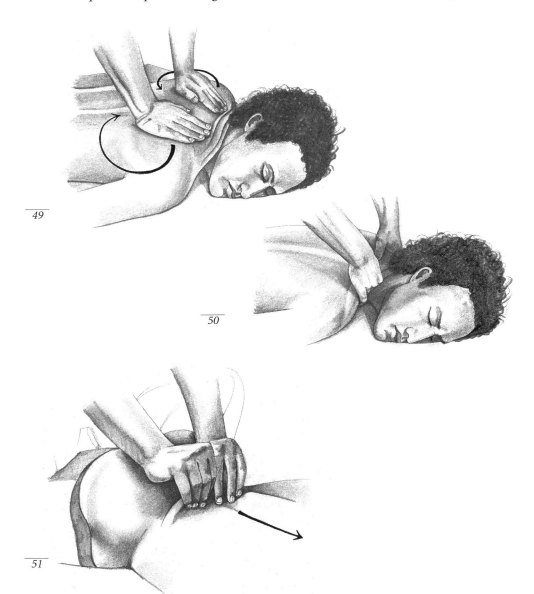

49

50

51

Massage of the back ends with a few fast rubbings up the back, with the thumbs fixed to either side of spine (see fig. 44). Then, moving from waistline to skull, lift the skin on both sides of the spine with your thumbs and forefingers (fig. 51); repeat this three times. The skin of a healthy person lifts easily. Massage a bit more in areas where it cannot be easily lifted. Sticking of the skin to the spine is a sign that the internal organ related to this part of the spine is not functioning well.

UPPER FRONT OF THE BODY

The Abdominal Area

This section of the full-body massage begins at the navel, the center of gravity and preservation of the body. According to Tantra and Ayurveda the navel is considered an important site in the body. Seventy-two thousand subtle nerves, or nadis, converge in this area. Through the navel a child is connected with the body of its mother before birth. All vital life-giving fluids flow from the mother's body into the child through this channel. Pranic energy also flows here, since the external nostrils of the child in the womb are clogged and inactive.

To prepare for abdominal massage, ask the recipient to turn over to a supine position, arms and feet stretched out and relaxed. To check the pulse, place the tips of your three middle fingers deep into the navel (fig. 52). The pulsation you feel is that of the nabhi marma. In a healthy person, this pulsation will feel strong under the middle finger. If the pulsation is not felt, ask the recipient to relax a bit, then soften your fingers and try again. If no pulsation is registered the second time, by any of the three fingers, the recipient most surely suffers from intestinal problems. This condition reflects a dislocation of the nabhi marma, which can happen by lifting weights, by pulling or pushing heavy objects, or by running or jogging.*

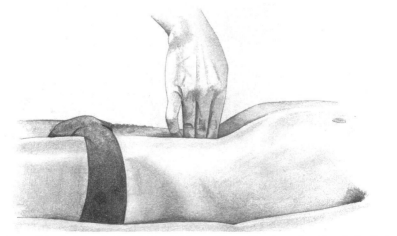

52

* Some naturopathic physicians in the West treat this condition with a type of suction device that aligns nerves.

Drip oil from your fingertips into the navel until the cavity can hold no more[*] and spread it using small clockwise movements (fig. 53). This stroke will excite the many lymph nodes located in this area. It also helps with the circulation of digestive fluids.

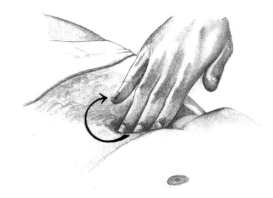

53

The Chest

Gently press the middle three fingers of both hands directly under the breast-bone (the xiphoid process), and then move your hands to the outer edge of the rib cage (fig. 54). On the recipient's right side is the liver, and on the left is the stomach. If pain is registered on either side, it indicates a problem in one of these two organs. Massage these sensitive areas carefully, with gentle, bearable pressure.

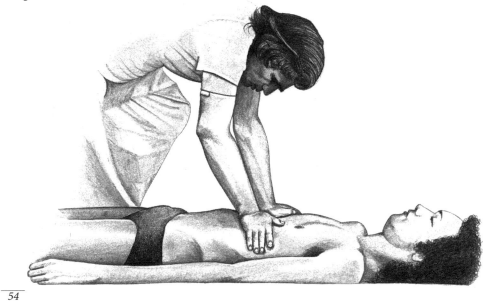

54

---

[*] There is an Indian folk belief about the shape of the navel. Gods in Indian iconography are always depicted as having deep navels. A deep navel is thought to bestow gentleness and good qualities on its beholder. People endowed with deep navels eat, sleep, and talk less than those who have navels of average depth. A protruding navel, according to folklore, is demonic and indicates a person who is eternally dissatisfied.

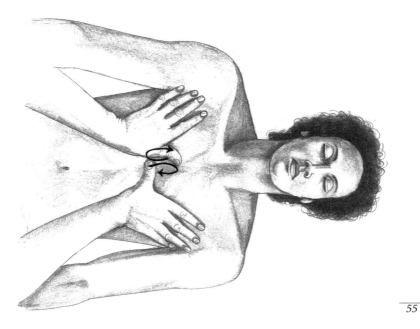

55

Moving upward, locate an important marma called hridayam, seated on top of the xiphoid process (fig. 55). Using both thumbs, rub and press on this marma with small circular movements. Pressure on this point brings relief to persons suffering from depression. Continue these small circular movements with the fingertips of both hands along the edges of the breastbone, going back and forth from the hridayam to the clavicle.

Apply oil to your hands and, using your middle three fingers, move from the breastbone in a semicircle toward the sides (fig. 56). While rubbing and pressing the muscles, lift and knead them also. This will help excite the fine nerves and blood capillaries, as well as strengthen the muscles and skin.

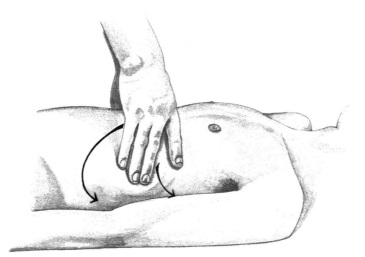

56

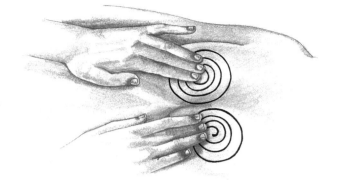

57

To massage the breasts, place the fingers of both hands on the outside of the rib cage, under the breasts. Make a spiral-like movement while gently rubbing and pressing the muscles around the nipple from all sides (fig. 57). Continue the spiral motion until the fingers reach the nipples. Repeat this procedure a few times, to produce heat and enhance circulation. This stroke helps give proper shape to the breasts.

To end the breast or chest massage, hold each nipple between your forefinger and thumb and pull very gently and lightly, but with enough strength to excite the fine capillaries of the vascular and nervous systems. This pulling motion increases the circulation of lymphatic fluid also, since a network of lymph nodes can be found all around the nipples. Men massaging women should skip the breast area and vice versa.

The Shoulder Girdle and Arms

Ask the recipient to sit in a comfortable cross-legged position in front of you. Locate the ansa marma at the front and back of the shoulders. Rub the front and back of the marma with both hands at once (fig. 58). Now select one side of the body and procede as follows.

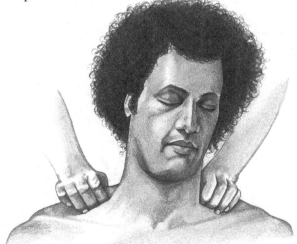

58

Locate the two important marmas in the underarm area, the lohitaksha and the apalapa marmas. Lohitaksha is found on the front of the underarm (fig. 59). Too much pressure on this point can make the whole arm temporarily weak or numb. However, gentle pressure, enough to feel the pulsation at the point, strengthens the locomotive power of the arm. Apalapa, located inside the underarm where the arm connects to the torso, is an important junction of nerves, blood capillaries, and lymph nodes. Working on this marma enhances circulation of lymphatic fluid. Apalapa marma is also a sensitive spot, and many people are ticklish here. Massage of this area provides courage and an inner resistance that helps one face the obstacles presented by the outside world.

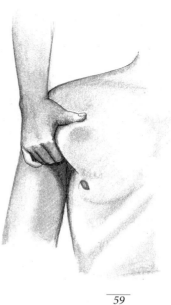

59

The Shoulder Blades

Sitting to the side of the recipient, ask the recipient to relax the arm by making slow and gently rhythmic movements with it, like those seen in Indian dance. Have the recipient bend the arm behind the torso, palm facing out (fig. 60). This position makes the shoulder blade prominent and accessible. Tap all the edges of the shoulder blade to bring relaxation and help increase the flow of energy.

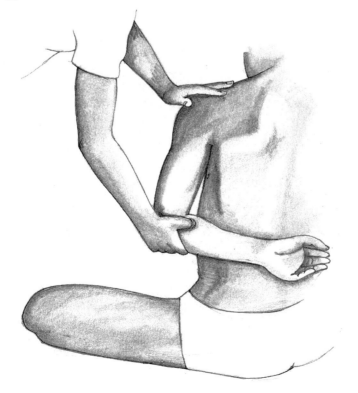

60

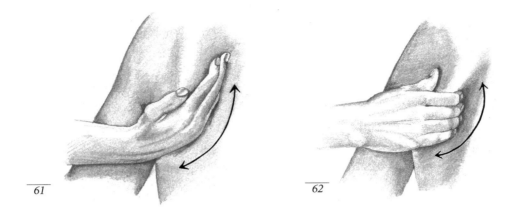

61

62

Apply oil to your hands and rub gently along the bony edge of the shoulder blade with the blade of your palm (fig. 61). Rub the flat part of the shoulder blades with your fingers.

The ansa phalak marma is located on the upper back in the middle of the shoulder blade, six fingerwidths from the spine. To palpate ansa phalak, make a circular movement with your fingers beneath the protruding shoulder blade (fig. 62). The point is usually painful to the touch. After rubbing this point on both sides to remove the tension and pain, go on to find the marmas in the neck area. Rub the two krikatikas marmas and the four posterior siramatrika marmas once again; also rub the two vidhuram marmas in the same way. Moving down from the neck to the back again, massage the shoulder blade with your palms and fingers, using an upward movement.

Now shift your position so you are seated in front of the recipient. Place the recipient's wrist on your shoulder. After a pause to take a few deep breaths, apply oil to your hands. Press the center of the armpit to locate the kakshadhara marma. Hold until the pulsation of the carotid artery is felt, then making small concentric circles, massage the area with moderate pressure. Although this point has been massaged previously, it is an important lymph node site that warrants being done again.

The Upper Arm

Assume a standing position and begin this portion of the full-body massage by tapping and pressing the muscles of the upper arm. After pressing, knead the muscles a bit and then apply oil to your hands and massage the upper arm. Locate the kakshadhara marma, situated in the armpit, four fingerwidths below the shoulder joint (fig. 63). This area can also be painful to the touch; massage in small, clockwise circles to release tension. Eight fingerwidths down the arm from the kakshadhara marma is the urvi marma (fig. 64), and four fingerwidths below urvi is the ani marma (fig. 65). Massage these in sequence, from the top down, in the same way as the other marmas, rubbing clockwise with the right hand and counterclockwise with the left.

Place your thumbs on the outside of the upper arm at the shoulder joint, with fingers on the inside of the arm. Massage downward with both hands in one long stroke, crisscrossing them at the elbow (fig. 66). Repeat this stroke quickly several times, alternating the starting position of your hands at the shoulder joint.

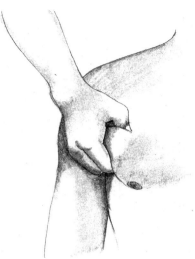

63

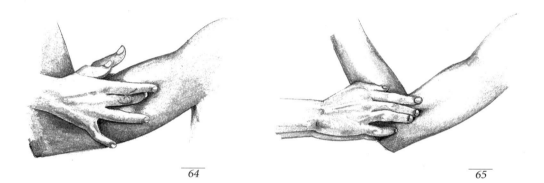

64

65

To end the massage of the upper arm, press the marma known as kurpara, situated in the hollow of the elbow. Place your fingers on both sides of the joint (fig. 67). Block the lateral kurpara while rubbing the medial kurpara with your middle finger. Then reverse your focus, and rub lateral kurpara while blocking the medial kurpara.

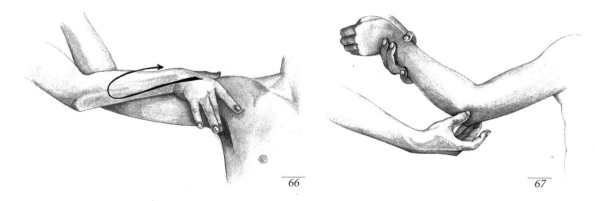

66

67

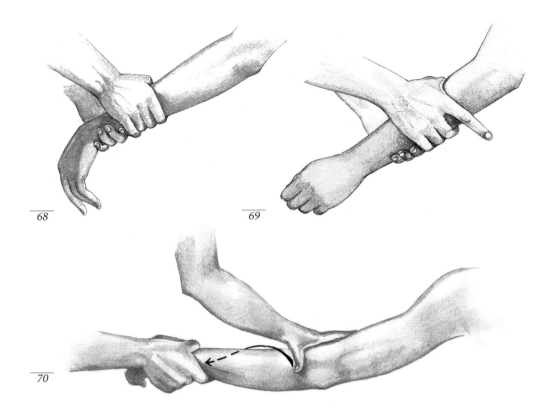

68

69

70

The Lower Arm

Remove pressure from the elbow marma and apply oil to your hands. Rub onto the lower arm, then knead with your thumb and forefingers (fig. 68).

While kneading, find and rub the indravasti marma, located in the middle of the inner arm (fig. 69). Continue rubbing back and forth on the lower arm until the oil is absorbed (that is, until no oil is visible). To massage the lower arm with both hands, cross your thumbs on the inside of the elbow, with hands wrapped around the arm. Move your hands rapidly in a crisscross fashion so that the thumbs move from inside to out as the palms approach the wrist (fig. 70). Repeat briskly to enhance circulation. Continue until the muscles are relaxed and loose.

The Wrists

There are two marmas situated on the wrist. Manibandha is found on the inside of the wrist exactly in the middle of the wrist joint; kurchshira aligns with manibandha just below the little finger (fig. 71). Apply oil to your thumbs and rub these marmas in the directions indicated (right hand rubs clockwise, left hand counterclockwise) for a few minutes. Then ask the recipient to rotate the wrist, creating hand postures like those seen in Indian dancing.

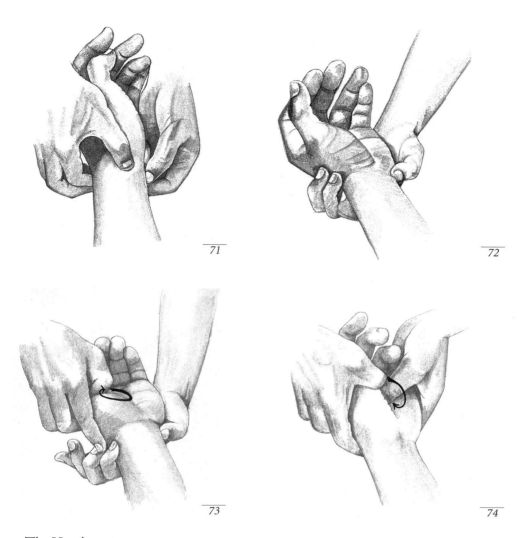

71

72

73

74

The Hand

For the first part of the hand massage, block the kurchshira marma below the little finger with your thumb (fig. 72). With your other hand, locate two marmas on the inner hand: one is kuruchcha, below the thumb in the middle of the mound of Venus, and the other is kshipra, below the index finger on the mound of Jupiter. While still blocking the kurchshira marma, rub these marmas one at a time (fig. 73). Release kurchshira marma and rub the middle region of the palm with your thumb. Then find and rub the talhridayam marma, located in the depression below the middle of the palm (fig. 74).

Apply oil to your thumbs and fingers in preparation for rubbing each finger joint. First massage the front and back of the palm with your whole hand, then massage each finger with your thumb and index finger. Locate the first joint of the index finger, under the heart line, and rub. Place the thumb of your support hand on the wrist to block the manibandha marma at the middle of the inner

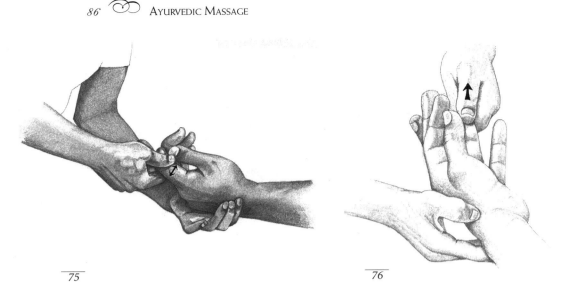

75

76

wrist joint. Then, starting with the first joint of the little finger, use your free thumb and index finger to articulate each joint, twisting the joint gently from side to side (fig. 75). Finally, pull each finger by force toward you (fig. 76). If the joint does not crack, rub the sides and try again. Pull as if you are milking a cow, moving slowly outward from the first joint toward the fingertips. This pulling stroke enhances circulation and supplies nutrients to the fingers. After all the fingers have been pulled, put a drop of oil on each nail (fig. 77).

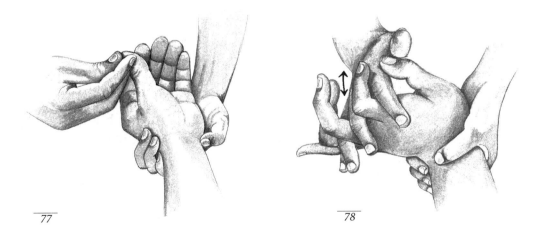

77

78

Massage the space between each finger near the first joint by interlocking the fingers of your free hand with those of the recipient (fig. 78). In closing, grasp the wrist with your thumb and index finger of your other hand. Press alternately on the front and back of the hand and fingers, working each joint. Then twist and pull the fingers once again. After pulling each finger, shake out your own hand.

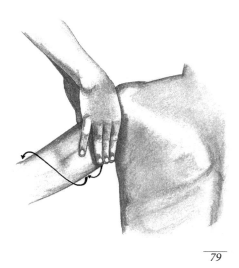

79

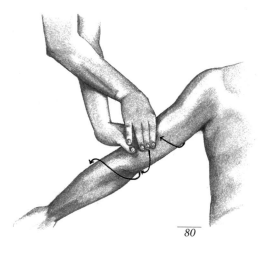

80

To end the upper torso massage, rub and squeeze the whole arm from shoulder to fingertip, making a crisscross movement with both hands (figs. 79–82). Use your palm and fingers to simultaneously press and pull. After squeezing as far as the fingertips, clap your hands.

Return to the instructions for massaging the shoulder girdle and arms (page 80). Beginning with the underarm, repeat steps for the opposite arm. When both arms have been massaged, move on to the massage of the head.

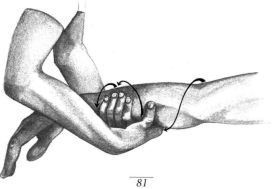

81

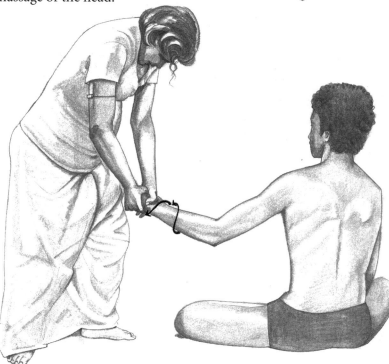

82

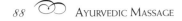
HEAD MASSAGE

If done properly, a head massage is in fact a massage of the entire body. Since the head is the center of the nervous system, a head massage calms the entire nervous system. The brain is the first organ to form in the process of fetal development. It is larger and heavier at birth than any other organ. (It normally takes three to six months for an infant to even hold and balance its head on its neck.)

The infant's "soft spot," or fontanelle, is a membrane-covered opening between the incompleted angles of the two parietal bones. Located at the top of the cranium over the midbrain, the fontanelle can be seen pulsating in a newborn. At the time of death, the vital force, or prana, leaves the body through one of the body's ten gates.* In the language of the yogis, the fontanelle is considered the tenth gate, or *brahmand*. This opening is meant to provide energy to the infant from the external environment. By six to nine months, the opening closes and this part of the skull becomes stiff and hard, like other bones. However, through constant practice of nada yoga (*pranava*), yogis can reopen it. (Nada yoga is the practice of chanting *Aum* in a low, almost inaudible voice. The sound vibrates the top of the cranium and resembles the hum of a bumblebee.) Yogis who leave the body through this gate do not take birth again.

Head massage, done very carefully with nourishing oils during the first six to nine months of life, is excellent for the infant's brain and eyesight. It protects the brain from dryness, which is constantly created in later years by thinking, imagining, and making decisions. When this opening closes, oil can no longer reach the brain. To ensure optimal functioning of an infant's brain, an Indian mother will keep a piece of cotton or linen soaked in oil on this soft area whenever possible.

Head massage done during the first nine months of life energizes the cerebrospinal fluid and strengthens the nervous system. The brahmand is thought to breathe and absorb pranic energy, solar radiation, and other forms of subtle energy present in the atmosphere. Oil, which also keeps the head cool, acts as a conductor of the energy available in the environment. According to yogic texts, this spot, located eight fingerwidths above the third eye, is believed to be the seat of the Self. It is the abode of consciousness during samadhi, a state of "conscious unconsciousness."†

Application of nourishing oils to this area helps to both calm and strengthen the brain and nervous system. When the oil is applied to the head of adults, it is

---

* The ten gates are the anus, genitals, mouth, two nostrils, two eyes, two ears, and the brahmand.

† Anatomically, the brahmand is the hollow space between the two cerebral hemispheres. This area is in the direct path of the mysterious kundalini (serpent power) that flows through the *sushumna*, the main subtle channel known to yogis.

absorbed by the hair roots; these in turn are connected with the nerve fibers that lead directly to the brain.

Oil strengthens the hair and removes dryness, which is responsible for brittle hair, premature balding, and many scalp disorders.

Head massage can be done anytime other than immediately after eating, during a fever, and under conditions when general massage is prohibited (see page 45). It is especially beneficial in the morning before bathing and in the evening after finishing the day's work. If done before retiring, it brings on deep sleep.

Massage of the forehead, application of pastes such as sandalwood* or *ubtan* (see page 129) or application of *malai* (skin of boiled milk) calms the system and generates a good feeling in the brain.

While the application of clay also cools the system, it creates a dryness and oil must be applied after the clay is removed.

Applying sandalwood paste to the forehead before meditation is a familiar practice in India among Hindus. By cooling the frontal lobe, the area of the brain most involved in thoughts and ideas, the paste helps to quiet the mind and invite a meditative state.

Massage of the temples improves eyesight and the power of concentration. It also creates a centered state.

Massage of the eyebrows relaxes the whole body and is especially beneficial for the eyes.

Massage of the forehead improves eyesight and one's power of concentration.

BENEFITS OF HEAD MASSAGE

- Increases the supply of fresh oxygen and glucose to the brain

- Relaxes the nervous system and eliminates the fatigue caused by mental stress and strain

- Improves circulation of that life-giving sap, the cerebrospinal fluid

- Increases the secretion of growth hormones and enzymes necessary for the growth and development of brain cells

- Increases the level of pranic energy inside the brain

- Cures dryness

- Retards hair loss, premature balding, and graying

For these reasons, head massage should be included in every daily schedule.

---

* To make sandalwood paste, rub a piece of sandalwood on a sandstone grinding stone. Add a few drops of water, a pinch of organic camphor powder, and a pinch of saffron. When the camphor and saffron dissolve in the water, mix into a fine paste and apply.

OILS FOR HEAD MASSAGE

∞ Sesame oil, extracted from black sesame seeds, is supposed to be the best oil for head and hair massage. It contains linoleic acid, one of the twenty-four enzymes that are very important for the brain.

∞ Mustard oil is also very nourishing for the brain and is especially good for the eyes. Quite popular in North India, it slows graying of the hair and strengthens the nerves. Mustard oil can sometimes irritate the skin of people not accustomed to using it. For this reason it is best mixed with sesame oil, which is neutral and does not irritate the skin.

∞ Coconut oil is particularly recommended because it is soothing to the body and is cooling compared to mustard or sesame oil. Because it is thought to promote long and lustrous hair, Indian women, especially those in Bengal, use coconut oil for head and hair massage.

∞ Several oils are especially good for the health of the hair. Amla oil nurtures and strengthens the hair. Bhringaraj oil slows graying. Shikakai oil promotes long and shiny hair. Sesame-almond oil with a small amount of sandalwood strengthens hair and memory. Jasmine is used for its delightful scent.

∞ Two other oils that aid memory are almond oil and brahmi oil.

∞ The oils known for their cooling effects are pumpkin seed, kahu, and coriander oils. Coriander oil is very cooling and should not be used in its pure form; mix it with other oils before using. This oil is especially beneficial for people with a hot head.

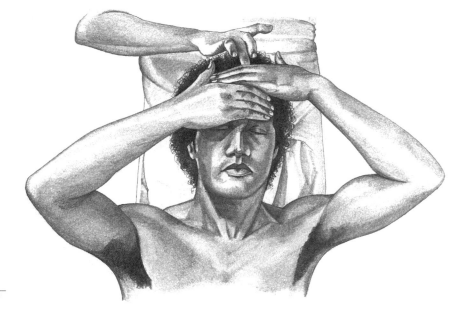

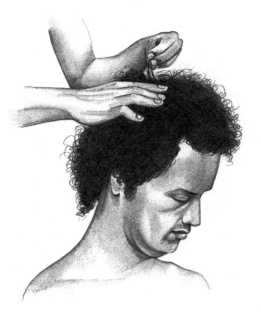

84

Many of these oils are used in combination for their benefits. Some common combinations are brahmi-amla, brahmi-amla-shikakai-bhringaraj, sesame-almond with jasmine, and almond-pumpkin-kahu.

Before beginning the head massage, it's important to first become familiar with three spots. Oil should be applied to these three spots and then spread onto the entire scalp.

1. The first spot is the fontanelle or brahmand, located eight fingerwidths up from the third eye (fig. 83). This is also called the adhipati marma.

2. The second spot is the part of the skull where the hairs gather in a swirl, or cowlick. This area, located twelve fingerwidths from the eyebrows, is also known as the crest. Even when Hindus shave their heads completely, they do not shave this area (fig. 84); the lock of hair, called *shikha,* is supposed to be a sign of a Hindu. The hairs are twisted clockwise and knotted together. The most important subtle nerve or nadi, the sushumna, which originates in the first chakra, bifurcates at the end of the medulla oblongata and its posterior aspect terminates at this spot. Hindus maintain a shikha to keep the energy working in this region. By twisting and knotting the hairs, fine capillaries connected with the roots are excited, which in turn improves the circulation of energy. This practice was once upon a time considered essential for practitioners of pranayama.

3. The third spot is behind the head, near where the neck meets the skull. Two very important marmas, called krikatikas, are located on either side of the last palpable vertebra. These will be discussed again in the section that follows.

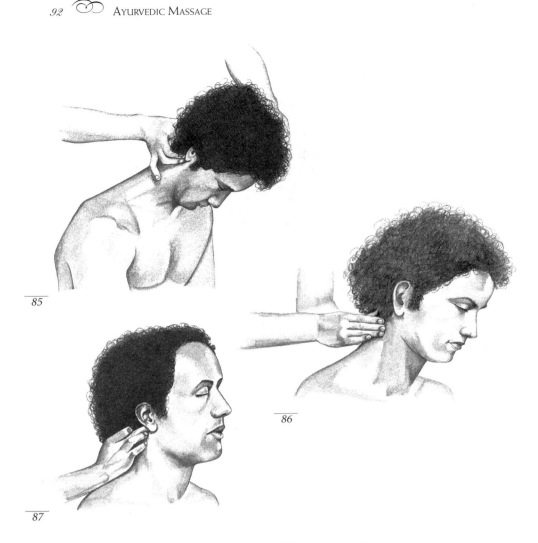

85

86

87

Massage of the Head and Neck

Have the recipient measure eight fingerwidths back from the eyebrows. This is the adhipati marma, which is situated on the coronal suture. Apply oil to that spot and spread it with the fingers of both hands to either side of the head. Rub it into the roots, distributing the oil uniformly.

Apply oil to the cowlick area, again using the fingers of both hands. Distribute the oil uniformly toward the temples. Finally, apply the oil with your fingers to the third spot, the hollow spot just below the skull.

Once the oil has been spread on all three areas, locate the krikatika marmas, on either side of the last palpable vertebra (fig. 85) and rub with a circular movement. Apply more oil to your fingers, if needed, and move on to find two sets of siramatrika marmas located on either side of the neck below the occiput (fig. 86). Once these four marmas are rubbed, move the fingers upward to the skull, behind the ears. The vidhuram marma is located in a depression behind the ear (fig. 87). Rub with oiled fingers as you have other marmas. Continue rubbing

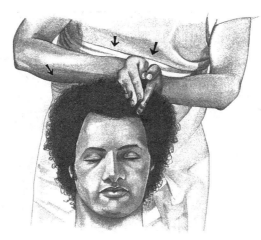

88

on the skull around the ear until your fingers reach the temples. Massage the neck once again, working with the areas of the krikatikas, siramatrika, and vidhuram marmas, before proceeding to the head.

The head massage starts with a gentle pounding of the head to excite the fine capillaries of the circulatory and nervous systems. To do this, bring the palms of your hands loosely together and, using an up-and-down motion, move from the crown to the base of the skull (fig. 88). Continue until you have pounded the entire skull area.

Then rub the skull toward the midline, moving your fingers from the base of the skull toward the cowlick. Twist the cowlick hairs clockwise, pulling them up with a gentle pressure (fig. 89). Rub the upper part of the skull. Then starting near the ears and temples, rub toward the fontanelle with both hands simultaneously. Twist a small lock of hair on the brahmand the same way you did the cowlick lock (fig. 90).

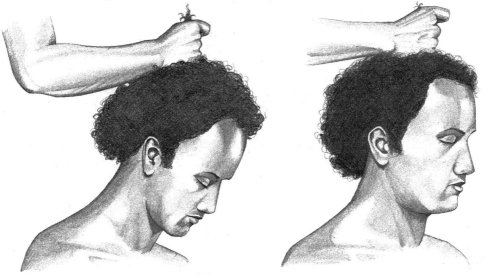

89   90

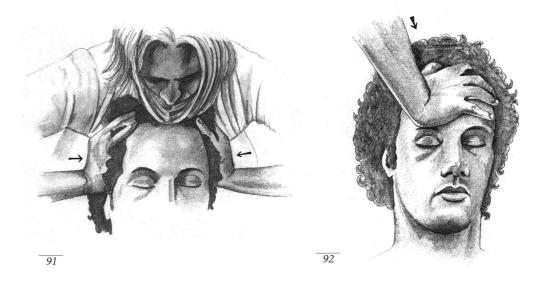

Take the head between your palms and apply bearable pressure all around (fig. 91). Apply the same pressure to the forehead (fig. 92). Hard pressure is actually desirable, if acceptable to the recipient.

To complete the head massage, pull small locks of hair on each of the three important spots once again: the fontanelle, the cowlick, and the hollow space below the skull.

MASSAGE OF THE EARS

Start this part of the massage with a gentle rubbing of the earlobes. As the most sensitive part of the ears, earlobes immediately warm up and get red in emotional states. They are connected to the brain by means of cranial nerves. In India it is believed that long, hanging earlobes are a sign of divinity and long life. Religious icons are depicted as having long, usually pierced earlobes. One particular sect of kundalini yoga practitioners pierced their ears and each wore a heavy earring. In ancient times both men and women pierced their ears and wore earrings. This practice is supposed to calm the mind, subdue the ego, and draw energy from the static electricity present in the environment. Pulling of the earlobes was a type of punishment given by a teacher to subdue a student's ego. People can often be seen pulling their earlobes when they don't want their words to be seen as egotistical.

The earlobes should be rubbed and pulled with oiled fingers. This is followed by a gentle rubbing and pressing of the ear cartilage itself and the folds of the outer ear. Finally, gently massage with an oiled finger the reachable area inside the ear, leading toward the eardrum.

MASSAGE OF THE FOREHEAD AND FACE

Stand behind the recipient and rest his or her head against your abdomen. Massage of the forehead starts on the midpoint of the forehead, where the sthapni marma is located (fig. 93). This point is in perfect alignment with the third eye, or sixth chakra. With thumbs at the hairline, place the fingers of both hands on the sthapni marma. Then rub the two upper sringataka marmas (fig. 94). Move your hands slowly out toward the temples and apply gentle pressure to the shankh marmas (fig. 95). Repeat this stroke a few times, ending massage of the forehead on the shankh marma.

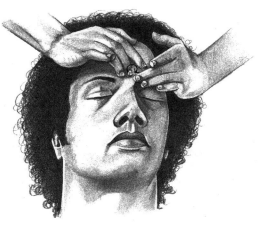

93

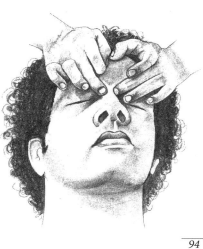

94

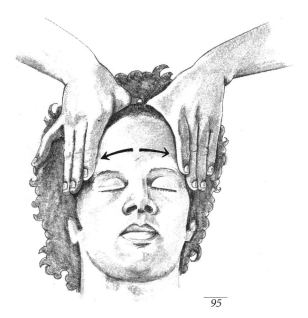

95

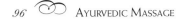

Return to the center of the forehead. Place your thumbs on the top edges of the eyebrows and your fingers below the eyebrows. Press along the upper edge of the eye sockets, moving your hands toward the temples (fig. 96). The avarta marmas are located near the end of the eyebrows. Once you palpate them, press gently with your thumbs (fig. 97). Then move your fingers toward the back of the head. Just above the ears, the utkshepa marmas can be found (fig. 98). Rub them gently.

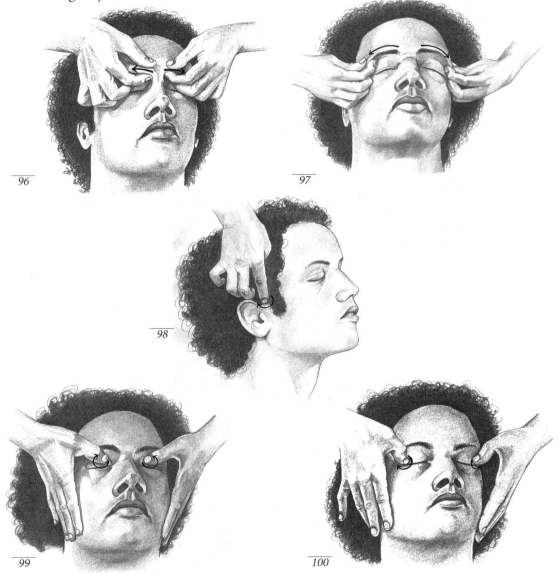

96

97

98

99

100

After making sure that the recipient is not wearing contact lenses, return your fingers to the center of the forehead. Gently press on each eyeball with your thumbs, moving toward the temples (fig. 99). Locate the apanga marma at the edge of the eye near the socket and gently press (fig. 100).

The massage of the cheeks is done without any oil. Lift each cheek gently with your fingers and thumbs (fig. 101). Press on the two lower sringataka marmas, above the lips (fig. 102) and below the chin (fig. 103), to release tension. After working these points, press on the chin with small, circular movements.

For lip massage, have the recipient apply almond oil or malai, the thin skin from boiled milk, directly to the lips. The practitioner should not massage the recipient's lips.

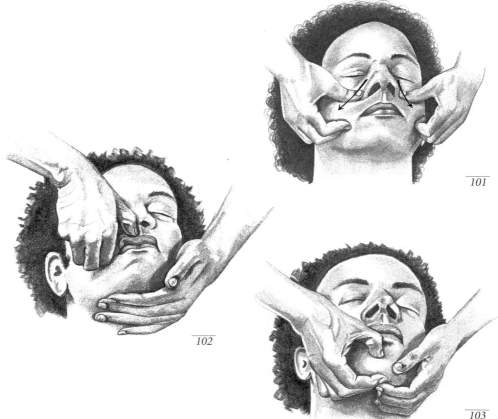

Gently massage the earlobes and outer ear for a few minutes. Then, with the recipient's head tilted to one side, pull the outer ear gently and place a drop of pure almond, sesame, or mustard oil* into the ear. Ask the recipient to open and close the jaw several times to allow oil to penetrate as you move the outer ear from side to side to widen the entry. Place a piece of cotton into the ear and repeat the same steps on the other ear. This treatment helps lubricate the area and helps the ear expell unwanted wax.

* This oil needs to be pure, cold-pressed, and unrefined. In the case of earaches, either warm the oil or use medicated oils prescribed by a physician. Sandalwood oil or mullein oil are an ideal addition to the medicated oil, unless other herbs are prescribed.

To treat the eyes, place one drop of rosewater[*] into each eye with an eyedropper. Not only is this cooling and cleansing, but the fragrance calms the body and strengthens the eye nerves and tissues. The final stroke for the head massage, and for the whole-body massage as well, is to gently rub the skull and tug on the lock of hair covering the fontanelle.

To signal the completion of the massage, clap your hands. Cover the recipient's whole body with a large towel or sheet, and ask the recipient to breathe deeply and relax.

---

[*] Be sure to use 100 percent natural rosewater distilled from rose petals. Do not use a synthetic. The rosewater should contain no alcohol, oil, or artificial fragrance.

ChapterSix

Therapeutic Massage

*I*n this chapter I will discuss diseases that can be cured or helped with Ayurvedic massage. While massage does not provide a complete therapeutic cure, it does help the organism receive nutrient material from within the body and expel toxins. It strengthens the immune system and helps the body move toward a speedy recovery. Certain ailments related to the muscles, ligaments, and nervous system can be completely healed through a good massage that employs healing oils prepared from herbs and other medicinal plants. In all cases, in order to remove illness massage must be combined with good food and healing medicines. In diseases caused by deranged vata, massage is the only remedy; in diseases caused by deranged pitta and kapha, it complements other healing methods.

Massage is an ideal remedy for pain. Figure 104 shows parts of the head as they relate to other body parts and/or symptoms of disease syndromes. Constant pain in one part of the head indicates a disorder in the body part corresponding to that area of the head. The massage practitioner should study this diagram and use it to refer his or her clients to a medical practitioner specializing in the body part the pain reflex indicates. The practitioner can provide massage as an adjunct to the medical doctor's program. A practitioner trained in Ayurveda can prescribe the appropriate Ayurvedic medicine and use massage, herbal remedies, gem powders, and proper diet to cure a client.

If the practitioner applies the teachings of color therapy and stores the massage oil in appropriately colored bottles in the sunlight and moonlight for 40 days and nights, the massage can yield miraculous results. After the 40 days have passed, keep the colored bottle in a cold and dry place. When you are ready

———
104

A. Pain here indicates tension and infections of the gums and teeth

B. Pain of the eyeball indicates overacidity

C. Pain of the eye socket indicates gastritis

D. Pain here indicates inflammation of the stomach

E. Pain here indicates ulcers

F. Pain here indicates disorders of the intestines

G. Pain here indicates disorders of the fallopian tubes

H. Pain here indicates kidney disorders

I. Pain here indicates disorders of the urinary tract

J. Pain here indicates neuralgia

K. Pain here indicates formation of cataract

L. Pain at the temple indicates disorders of the brain and spinal nerves.

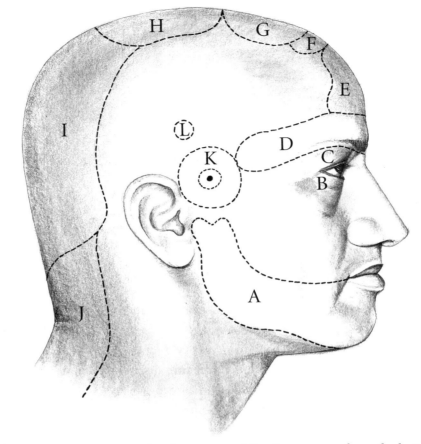

to give a massage, remove only what you need for the massage from the bottle. Since the oil is cold, place the amount you are using in a cup and sit it in hot water for a few minutes.

Almond oil is an especially good base for making oils in color therapy. A full range of glass-bottle colors, such as red, orange, yellow, green, light and deep blue, and violet, are used to store oil being used for different conditions. To the almond oil you may add other oils, depending on your needs.

CONDITIONS AND METHODS FOR TREATMENT

General Weakness

Invalids, seniors, and underdeveloped children can be helped by the following therapeutic mixture. Combine equal parts of cold-pressed black sesame seeds or yellow mustard seeds with either olive, almond, or a fish oil, such as cod liver oil.* Keep the mixture in an orange glass bottle for 40 days, then store in a cold,

---

* If fish oil is not available, oil extracted from the fat of water birds can be used.

dry place. When this oil is stored in an orange bottle it is especially beneficial for a male client; for a female, a yellow glass bottle is preferred, unless she has a tendency toward depression or pessimism. Yellow may be a depressive for those who have a tendency toward depression.

Sprains or Dislocated Bones

According to the *Sushruta Samhita,* the symptoms of dislocation are an inability to extend, flex, or rotate a limb, as well as extreme pain and intolerance to touch. Anyone with a dislocation must first have the bone reset before receiving any sort of massage. A dislocated joint should not be shaken but rather should be kept at rest. Cold lotions, washes, and medicinal plasters[*] can be applied to the joint until it can be reset. It can also be kept covered with a linen cloth soaked in oil, ghee, or clarified butter. After the bone has been returned to its proper place by someone skilled in this art, the joint can be massaged with one of the following therapeutic mixtures.

MUSTARD OIL AND IODEX

> $1/2$ cup of mustard oil
> $1/2$ teaspoon of iodex

Add iodex, an allopathic formula made with iodine, to the mustard oil. Mix well, shake, and apply to the affected area.

MUSTARD OIL COMBINATION

> 2 tablespoons of mustard oil
> 1 teaspoon powdered turmeric
> $1/2$ teaspoon iodex
> 10 drops mint oil
> 30 drops almond oil

Mix ingredients together, shake, and apply to the affected area.

For either combination, rub gently for about 30 minutes and then apply a warm water bottle to the area for another 45 minutes. The application of a strip of cloth coated with a clay paste can also be beneficial. Both combinations should be stored in a green glass bottle.

---

[*] Cold lotions can take the form of base oils mixed with essential oil of mint, eucalyptus, wintergreen, or camphor, ideally cold and stored in a green bottle. Washes can include water in which herbs, such as oregano or fenugreek seed, or neem, eucalyptus, lemon, or marigold leaves, have been boiled (oregano seeds must boil 4 to 5 minutes). Plasters can be made of soft clay or the following herbal mix: combine $1/2$ teaspoon turmeric, $1/2$ cup wheat flour, 4 teaspoons water, 6–10 drops oil (preferably mustard), and a pinch of salt. Put plaster onto cloth strips and apply to the dislocated joint.

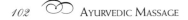

Arthritis

According to Ayurveda, arthritis is caused by deranged or aggravated vata, also referred to as vayu. Vayu diseases have their origins in the large intestine and are related to unabsorbed iron in the intestines. To alleviate this condition, Ayurveda prescribes enemas (basti) with oil, consisting of ½ cup warm sesame oil, or a decoction enema, in which herbs are soaked or boiled in sesame oil or another liquid medium.* Fasting on warm water—1 to 2 quarts per day—also helps arthritic pain, which is caused by poor circulation in the joints due to deranged vayu. Vata diseases usually attack an organism in old age because old age is the time of vata. Alfalfa, fenugreek, or castor-root tea taken before bedtime can be helpful. Swallowing a small, peeled garlic clove followed by a ball of beeswax, the size of a garbanzo bean, for 40 days has also shown to be effective for arthritis. Turmeric, taken internally or used externally in a massage oil, is very helpful also. Fenugreek seeds are beneficial and can be boiled in mustard or sesame oil, or simply mixed in the oil before massage. Alfalfa and fenugreek sprouts should be eaten in salads by arthritis sufferers.

Before giving a massage to someone with arthritis, the practitioner should give a fomentation—a treatment with a warm, moist substance. This is done by soaking linen cloths in warm water and applying them to the affected area for 3 minutes. Then apply cloths soaked in cold water for 1 minute. Repeat the warm water fomentation, then massage the area with the following therapeutic mixture.

Combine 2 tablespoons each of olive and mustard oil,† 1 tablespoon fenugreek seed oil,‡ ¼ teaspoon turmeric powder, and 10 drops each of wintergreen, eucalyptus, and mint oil. Shake mixture well and store in a yellow glass bottle. If there is not time to cure the oil in sunlight for 40 days, 1½ teaspoons of almond or sesame oil that already has been cured by the sun in a yellow bottle may be added to the mixture.

After massaging the affected areas for 5 to 10 minutes with this mixture, tie a cloth coated with clay paste (either healing clay from France or potter's clay) onto the area and leave for 40 minutes. If this prescription is followed daily for 40 days, it will bring relief to arthritis sufferers.

---

* One type of decoction basti can be made using an equal amount of the herbs that make up triphala (haritaki [*Terminalia chebula*], bibhitaki [*Terminalia belerica*], and amla) or triphala powder, which is easily available. Boil 1 teaspoon of triphala powder in ¼ cup of water until water is reduced to half. Strain and add liquid to 1 cup of preheated oil. The oil is necessary so as not to dry out the colon and further aggravate vata. Allow to cool before using.

† Sesame oil may be used if these oils are not available.

‡ Fenugreek seed oil is not available in stores. It can be made by boiling 1 tablespoon of seeds in ½ cup of sesame or mustard oil. When the seeds turn black, filter the oil and store it for future use.

Rheumatism

Rheumatism involves pain in the bones, joints, muscles, tendons, or nerves. However, most of the pain is experienced in the joints because they are important areas for movement. Since joints are sites where blood vessels must twist and turn, it is a natural place for waste materials to accumulate and become clogged. Improper eating creates toxins that, after digestion, are transmitted to the blood; these toxins in turn become overly acidic and impure. As digestion becomes poor, and indigestion and constipation set in, vayu (bodily gases) becomes deranged. In rheumatism, vayu gets blocked by a mucuslike coating known as ama, which is produced in the intestines. In Ayurveda this poisonous ama is called *aamvish*. The blocked vayu enters the circulatory system, causing problems with muscles, joints, and nerves. Like arthritis, rheumatism is mainly a vata disorder and medicated enemas are the treatment of choice. This procedure alleviates both constipation and hyperacidity. Oil enemas should be avoided by those who suffer from chronic indigestion, hypoacidity, chronic cough, breathlessness, diarrhea, diabetes, or anemia. They also should not be given to the elderly or those under seven years of age. For rheumatic sufferers who fall into the above categories, decoction enemas, in which herbs are either boiled or soaked in water, may be given providing the recipient does not have a fever, chest cold, paralysis, heart pain, or severe abdominal pain. (People with diarrhea should not be given any kind of enema.)

Several other remedies have proven beneficial with rheumatism. Alfalfa tea may be taken at bedtime. Castor oil, which is antirheumatic and a natural pain reliever, acts as a laxative and can be taken with a cup of ginger tea.* Garlic is also antirheumatic and its oil can be used in massage to relieve joint pain. Rheumatic pain is caused by toxins deposited near the joints; as long as these deposits are not removed, health cannot be restored. It is essential to achieve a balance in the body chemistry. This can be done in many ways, such as through sweating, a cleansing massage, or a hard massage and an enema. Sweating can be induced by fomentation and is an effective means of cleansing the body of toxins. Steam baths or saunas are also powerful tools for removing toxins. These elimination methods should ideally follow a massage. While any edible oil may be used, the following oils are suggested.

- Olive oil (preferably in which garlic cloves have been charred)
- Mustard oil (preferably in which garlic cloves have been charred)

---

* To make ginger tea, cut a half-inch piece of fresh ginger into small pieces. Place ginger in 1 cup of water and boil until water is reduced to half. (If you choose, you may boil ¼ cup of milk along with the water.) Add ¼ teaspoon of black tea leaves and serve with Sucanat.

- Cold-pressed black sesame seed oil ($^1/_2$ cup) with fenugreek seeds (1 teaspoon)
- Any oil in which fenugreek seeds have been charred
- Babuna (chamomile) oil (can be mixed with castor oil)
- Mahanarayana oil (can be mixed with castor oil)
- A mixture of babuna and mahanarayana oils
- Any oil from a blue, yellow, or green bottle

Following the massage, it is beneficial to apply a paste made of ground fenugreek seeds to a strip of cloth and tie the cloth around the afflicted joint.

Neurasthenia

Often found in people of vata temperament, this disease is mental and is caused by weakness of the brain and nervous system. Patients often complain of backaches and pain, especially around the waist. Sometimes they experience a burning sensation in the head area and their eyes or ears become red. As a result of weakened blood capillaries, their minds are influenced and they lose the power to make decisions. They become fickle minded and lose confidence and faith in themselves, as well as in others. People suffering from neurasthenia think negatively about themselves and others, and sometimes have feelings of paranoia or persecution. Constant worry, anxiety, and restlessness cause, as well as nurture, this condition. Under extreme conditions patients can act psychotic and even be suicidal. Love and caring attention can provide relief to the constant tension they experience. Excessive sexual indulgence, futile fantasizing, and the use of hallucinogenic drugs or other drugs that weaken the nervous system also cause this disease.

In addition to regular psychotherapy, massage is a must for these patients. They need to relax and strengthen their nervous, digestive, and circulatory systems. Massage can help them enjoy deep sleep and thus reduce their restlessness. Through constant worry and tension, their digestion and assimilation become impaired. Good diet can be beneficial.

Foods that can help strengthen their systems include milk, yogurt, salads, fruits, vegetables, and whole wheat bread. Green vegetables, such as spinach, fenugreek leaves and sprouts, coriander, mint, and amaranth leaves are beneficial; leeks, carrots, cabbage, and turnips are also good. Chlorophyll from green vegetables helps the metabolism of those suffering from neurasthenia, and organic raisins—due to their laxative quality and high glucose content—can help clean their systems. Pulpy vegetables, such as zucchini and other types of squash, are also beneficial.

Massage that includes hard rubbing, pinching, squeezing, and tapping is helpful. The ideal massage oil for this condition is an equal combination of pumpkin seed oil and sandalwood oil. Applying sandalwood paste (see footnote on page 89 for recipe) to the forehead, temples, and earlobes or to the whole head, including the crown, sides, and back, aids in curing this condition. After the massage, the patient may take a sunbath with leaves and twigs covering the head. The twigs and leaves allow the body to absorb the sunlight and heat without disturbing its electromagnetic field.

Following the massage, the neurasthenia patient should take a bath. In winter, the water should be lukewarm; in summer, the bath should be cold or slightly below room temperature. Cold water strengthens the nerves. Bathing in a river when the water is not too cold is also helpful. Massage of the back and spine can be done using alternately warm and cold oil. At the end of the massage, a hot water bottle can be applied to the waist region for five or ten minutes. This treatment can be followed by a good rubbing with a cold towel. Alternating heat with cold strengthens the nervous system and accelerates the production of growth hormones. Regular morning walks before sunrise are effective in bringing the body chemistry into balance and also provide relief. In addition, sheets of gold leaf taken with honey can be ingested as an effective nerve tonic.[*]

High Blood Pressure

Luxurious living; excess weight; laziness; inertia; eating too much fat, oil, butter, and ghee; smoking; and drinking are the main causes of high blood pressure. High cholesterol, eating hot spices and pickles, and taking in rich foods—including excess nuts such as almonds and cashews, when your system has insufficient digestive fire to process them—cause blocks in the circulatory system. This forces the heart to work harder in order to pump blood through the constricted capillaries. Lifestyle changes must be made if a complete cure is to be obtained. Eating only as much as one can easily digest and engaging in physical labor, which increases the digestive fire, enhances circulation, and strengthens the nerves, are good habits to develop. Cholesterol levels can be lowered by fasting on zucchini and ginger soup (1 level teaspoon of freshly grated ginger) for 2 weeks, followed by a 1-week fast on fresh juice—either papaya, honeydew melon, or carrot. No less than 3 quarts of juice should be taken per day. Each evening during the juice fast, one should take a glass of warm milk with a pinch of saffron and a few dates to sweeten, if desired.

Massage, in conjunction with lifestyle changes, is a most effective remedy for high (and low) blood pressure, and it should be performed regularly. Almond oil or black sesame seed oil from a yellow bottle should be mixed with an equal

---

[*] Although silver leaf is easily found in Indian shops, gold leaf is not as accessible. For a mail order source, see the Appendix. Take one leaf of pure gold leaf with 1 teaspoon of honey.

portion of mustard or olive oil for this treatment. Half a teaspoon of essential oil of rose may be added for a fragrant scent and to make the oil soothing to the heart. Massage with sandalwood oil mixed with black sesame oil from a yellow bottle is also very effective for patients with high blood pressure.

People with high (or low) blood pressure should never have the head massaged. When giving a full body massage, the practitioner should start working from the feet to help connect the recipient to the physical body, then continue massage from the waist and massage the torso. A foot massage before going to bed is very beneficial for blood pressure conditions. Gentle, light pressure applied over an extended time should be given, in a cozy environment. For increased effectiveness, the juice of half a lemon that has been placed in a yellow bottle in the sun for an hour can be added to 1/4 cup of the oil mixtures used for the massage.

The patient can also drink lemon juice and water that has been stored in yellow bottles. No more than 1/2 cup should be taken at once. To make enough for 6 doses, mix the juice of 1 1/2 lemons with 3 cups of water and take 1/2 cup every 2 hours.

In India, wearing a *rudraksha* bead necklace (a necklace made of *Elaeocapus ganitrus* berries) is a well-known cure for high blood pressure. If a full necklace is not available, some rudraksha beads strung on a red thread should be worn around the neck. A morning walk, as well as massage of the feet before retiring, should become part of the patient's daily routine.

Low Blood Pressure

This condition is caused by insufficient nutrients in the body due to poor blood circulation. Foods that assist in the production of blood should be eaten, and methods that remove toxins from the blood should be adopted. Massage is an effective method of purifying and stimulating the circulatory system. It also strengthens the digestive system and helps the body, much like exercise does.

For low blood pressure patients, hard but bearable pressure should be applied. Dairy foods should be avoided or not taken until 3 to 4 hours after eating fish, eggs, or other nonvegetarian food. Servings of salads, fruits, and fruit juices should be increased. Fasting on fresh juice, such as papaya, carrot, mango, or honeydew melon, for 1 week is very helpful.

Massage with 1 tablespoon of sesame oil or almond oil, kept in a yellow bottle, combined with 1/4 cup of either mustard or olive oil is beneficial. To this can be added a little lemon juice that has been kept in the sun for 1 hour in a yellow bottle. Sandalwood oil or rose oil can lend a nice fragrance and also soothe the heart. Breathing exercises, early morning walks, and communing with nature can be helpful. For those who can tolerate milk, a glass of warm milk with 10 to 12 saffron threads and 1 teaspoon of almond oil at bedtime is beneficial. Regular organic raisins and munnaquka raisins, made from large dried grapes, should be eaten a few times each day.

Patients with low blood pressure should massage their feet each night before retiring with beeswax cream (see page 134). Full-body massage reduces the sinking feeling in the heart and the depression that often is a main difficulty in low blood pressure. The use of rudraksha beads is also beneficial.

Sciatica

Sciatica is a condition often found in people of vata temperament in which the sciatic nerve, which runs from the lumbar spine to the bottom of the instep and toes, becomes stuffed or pressurized with enraged vata. This condition sometimes deprives the lower extremities of locomotion. Pain is experienced in the buttocks, the back of the leg and ankle, and sometimes in the waist area. Extended rubbing on the sciatic point near the ankle (the gulpha marma) with small circular movements can bring relief. Applying a hot water bottle to the pain site at the hip joint, waist, thigh, or ankle is also beneficial. While rubbing the pain site for an extended period of time produces heat, it is not enough heat. Having a massage in the sunlight, or taking a sunbath following the massage, would help.

The massage practitioner should use rubbing, kneading, and deep pressing techniques on the painful spots. Add ¼ teaspoon of finely grated and charred nutmeg to ¼ cup of cured massage oil from a yellow bottle. Filter and apply this mixture to the painful spots. Also, a paste of powdered fenugreek seeds and water placed on a strip of cloth can be applied to the afflicted area. For massage of the whole body, the practitioner should use a mixture of ¼ cup sesame oil from a yellow bottle, and 2 tablespoons mahanarayana oil or 1 tablespoon arnica oil. To this may be added 1 tablespoon of mustard oil in which fenugreek seeds have been charred. Eating fenugreek sprouts, olive oil, and garlic in salads is also beneficial.

Paralysis

Often an aftereffect of deranged vata, this condition either affects the legs, arms, and head in succession, or extends all over the body and deranges all the dhatus. Massage is the only technique to bring a numb or lifeless area back to life. Application of almond oil from a yellow bottle is very beneficial in paralysis. Orange juice and milk (taken at least 1 hour apart) are both good for this condition.

Several daily massages over a long period of time are necessary to bring relief. Each day the practitioner should use a different oil combination as shown in the list below. Note that the main oil—the first oil listed in each entry—should already be cured in a yellow bottle.

Day 1:	1 tablespoon of almond oil mixed with $\frac{1}{4}$ cup of mustard oil
Day 2:	$\frac{1}{4}$ cup of almond oil mixed with 1 tablespoon of fish oil
Day 3:	$\frac{1}{8}$ cup of almond oil mixed with $\frac{1}{8}$ cup of olive oil
Day 4:	$\frac{1}{8}$ cup of almond oil mixed with $\frac{1}{8}$ cup of mahanarayana oil
Day 5:	$\frac{1}{2}$ cup of almond oil mixed with 1 tablespoon of oil from the fat of a water bird
Day 6:	Begin cycle again with Day 1

The practitioner should be able to observe which mixture provides the most relief, and then use that mixture more often. Alternating hot and cold massage* enhances circulation. A good vegetarian diet and sunbathing aid in a quick recovery. Gem powders that nourish the dhatus also should be used.† If the patient is weak or elderly, almond oil from a red bottle could be added to the base massage oil, or to salads for eating.

Polio

Basically a disease contracted by children, polio is caused by poor circulation which in turn may have been caused by conditions such as viral infections. Deranged vayu causes atrophy of muscles and bones. Massage with medicated oils, preferably done at least four times daily in sunlight or under an orange light, can help cure polio. Following the massage, the patient should sit in a tub of hot water for 3 minutes, then apply hot- and cold-water compresses alternately for a minute or so each for 20 minutes. The afflicted area should be massaged with a mixture of equal amounts of fish oil and almond or sesame oil from a yellow, orange, or red bottle. A mixture of mahanarayana oil and black sesame seed oil, kept in a yellow, orange, or red bottle, can also be applied to the area. The rest of the body should be massaged with regular massage oil, such as almond, sesame, mustard, or olive.

Patience is an essential ingredient on the part of both the practitioner and the patient, as months of massage may be required before improvement is noticed. Massage done 4 times a day and the use of garlic and fenugreek seeds in food may help, but to a limited degree. Complete recovery is a miracle, which does not happen with every patient.

Insomnia

According to the *Sushruta Samhita*, insomnia is caused by aggravated vata or pitta (wind or bile). Insomnia may also be brought on by an aggrieved state of mind, loss of vital fluid, or a hurt or injury. Measures that nurture sleep must be

---

* Massage done with warm hands and oil or cold hands and oil.

† Lapis lazuli powder, blue saphire powder, and tourmaline oxide are beneficial for paralysis.

put in place, such as massaging the feet before retiring, anointing the body,* and massaging the head with pumpkin seed oil, kahu oil, or an equal mixture of the two. Massaging the body softly and gently, using cleansing pastes, shampooing, and eating a diet of cakes and pastry, milk, and grapes would help the patient recover quickly, as would a soft and pleasant bed. This condition, if allowed to continue for a long time, can cause a nervous breakdown. The bodily rhythms get disturbed by acting contrary to the laws of nature. Going to bed late and getting up late; having an uninteresting job; keeping irregular living habits; anxieties, stresses, and strains—these are the main causes of insomnia.

Most often, people who work less with their bodies than their minds suffer from this ailment. Mental fatigue causes a disturbance in the nervous system, preventing relaxation or sleep. Smoking tobacco, eating late at night, reading exciting literature, and living in an enclosed apartment can cause insomnia, as can heart palpitations and feelings of guilt or excitement.

The drone of an Indian musical instrument called a tamboura, or any drone providing it is not electronic, provides complete cure for this condition without any drugs. Usually this music is most effective if played while the patient is receiving a relaxing massage, whether to the full body, foot, or head.

Charaka, author of the *Charaka Samhita*, gives a vivid description of sleep:

> When the active self of the person,
> tired in body and mind,
> Loses touch with his worldly affairs,
> sleep comes to him.
> All pleasures and pains, health and disease,
> vitality and weakness, growth and decay,
> wisdom and ignorance, even life and death,
> Come to us through sleep.

When we awake from a night's sleep feeling that sickness has crept inside of us during the night, our sleep can be categorized as produced by:

- Tamas (inertia, heaviness)
- Increased mucus in the body
- Physical and mental strain
- Untimely sleep
- Disease

According to the *Sushruta Samhita*, sleep is the elusive energy of the all-pervading deity and naturally has its influence over all created beings. The kind

---

* Such as annointing oneself with beeswax cream, sandwood oil, rose oil, or jasmine oil.

of sleep that sets in when the sensory nerves (sensation-carrying nerves) of the body are choked by *sleshma* (mucus), which abounds in the quality of tamas, is known as tamasic sleep. This is the sleep that produces unconsciousness at the time of dissolution or death. A man of tamasic temperament sleeps both night and day; one of rajasic temperament sleeps either in the night or day; the eyelids of one of sattvic temperament are never visited by sleep before midnight. Those with weak kapha and aggravated vayu, or those suffering from physical or mental troubles, get little sleep, if any at all. Their sleep is of the vaikarika or delirious type, meaning much disturbed. Such persons may only get sleep when exhausted, which is the only time they can cease thinking of their affairs.

Sleep in the daytime is forbidden in all seasons of the year according to Ayurveda, except in summer, in the case of infants and the elderly, those who have overindulged sexually, and chronic alcoholics. Men suffering from the loss of fat, mucus, or blood, or from indigestion, are also exceptions; however, they should only sleep for one *muhurta* (48 minutes). Also, those who have been awake during the late hours may sleep for half of the time they have been awake. Daytime sleep aggravates all three doshas of the body and brings on conditions like coughs, asthma, catarrh, heaviness, aching or lassitude in the limbs, fever, and loss of appetite.

Sleep naturally comes at nighttime because of the position of the Earth and the effect of gravity. This sleep is Divine. It cleans garbage from the mind through dreams; it improves one's health, stamina, vitality, and wisdom; and improves one's knowledge of the Self. In this natural sleep, the body reorganizes itself. Only this sleep is genuine. Other types of sleep are caused by the increase of tamas and should be avoided.

Early morning walks, massage of the back and head during the day, and massage of the feet and head before retiring all help insomnia. The practitioner should be someone who is liked or revered by the patient. (Self-massage in insomnia cases is not very helpful.) Thirty minutes after a massage the patient should take alternately hot and cold baths or showers, each only 2 minutes in duration. Before bathing, the patient's head should be rinsed with room-temperature water and wrapped in a wet towel.

Bronchitis

This condition is most common is people with kapha constitutions. Ayurveda recommends therapeutic vomiting as an effective cure because it removes excess mucus from the body and brings relief to the system. Massage of the rib cage and chest region with oil from a yellow bottle mixed in equal amounts with black sesame or mustard oil is helpful. Sesame oil combined with 10 drops of eucalyptus oil can also bring relief.

Chapter Seven

Massage During Pregnancy

$\mathcal{P}$regnancy is a special condition. During this time a woman goes through a series of changes, both in her metabolism and in her mind. Under the best of circumstances she will have made her musculature flexible and supple before pregnancy through exercises such as yoga asanas and pranayama, through massage, and through the study of nutrition. But even if she has not prepared for this significant event in advance, the first three months of pregnancy may be devoted to this end. Techniques of relaxation and meditation should also be learned since they will enhance serenity, which is necessary to becoming a good mother. During pregnancy a woman experiences an intimate connection between her body and mind. She also must keep harmony inside of her body and mind.

The practices of massage, yoga asanas, pranayama, and meditation affect the entire organism and promote optimum health of both body and mind. They unify the physical, emotional, and spiritual sides of a pregnant woman, thus providing a better chemical environment for the growth of the child inside. These practices also enhance the likelihood of a quick recovery after childbirth.

ABDOMINAL/SPINAL MASSAGE WITH ASANAS: FIRST THREE MONTHS

Good massage, accompanied by specific asanas such as *matsyasana* (fish pose), *shashakasana* (rabbit pose), *hamsasana* (swan's pose), and *ushtrasana* (camel pose), as well as pranayama exercises, will strengthen the abdominal muscles. This combination of practices will help the expectant mother carry the baby and will assist in the proper development of the fetus. The abdominal muscles play a major role during delivery by pushing the child from the womb. During the first three months, the massage practitioner should concentrate on the abdomen and the spine. It is the spinal massage and yoga asanas that will increase the spine's flexibility during this time. A strong spine is essential because it helps the pregnant woman carry the extra weight; it also prevents the drooping shoulders that often can be seen during pregnancy. Massage also strengthens the nerves, and a properly functioning nervous system helps the fetus develop and grow. *Paschimottanasana* (forward bend) and *surya namaskar* (sun salutation) are ideal asanas to practice during the first three months of pregnancy. These poses help relieve the extra strain put on the back and pelvic muscles caused by the weight of the growing fetus.

Oil massage of the abdominal and spinal regions should be performed in the following order: First the practitioner should concentrate on the pelvis, then the spine, and finally on the abdominal muscles. Flexibility in the pelvic region helps to promote an easy childbirth, while massage of the back muscles strengthens the back area and helps the mother hold the extra weight of the child. Squatting and crossed-legged postures of all types help strengthen the pelvis; they also provide relaxation, promote flexibility, and facilitate an easy delivery.

BACK MASSAGE WITH RELAXATION EXERCISES: LAST SIX MONTHS

After the third month of pregnancy all strenuous yogic asanas, or ones that require the manipulation of muscles, are discontinued. In northern India, women do not do any yogic postures after the third month of pregnancy except gentle bending or squatting exercises. The only practices that may be continued up to the time of delivery and beyond are the five poses already mentioned (matsyasana, shashakasana, hamsasana, ushtrasana, paschimottanasana), surya namaskar, massage, pranayama and relaxation techniques, and meditation.

According to the *Sushruta Samhita,* a woman should avoid the following: all kinds of physical labor, fasting, sleeping in the daytime, late nights, indulgence in grief and fright, travel by carriages, sexual intercourse, and voluntary retention of any natural urges.

Anything that might adversely affect the position of the baby in the womb should also be carefully avoided. Back massage—that is, massage of the pelvis, spine, and back muscles—should be emphasized at this time. This massage may be complemented by simple deep-breathing exercises (pranayama) or other relaxation practices.

There are many varieties of pranayama, or controlled breathing practices, that are prescribed to nonpregnant yoga practitioners. Pregnant women should do a type of pranayama known as *bhastrika* (bellows breath) or an easier practice known as *surya bhadan*. Surya bhadan begins by inhaling with the right nostril for the count of two, then holding for a count of eight, and exhaling for a count of two. Pregnant women should be sure not to hold the breath longer than is comfortable. The practice should be relaxing and gentle.

Deep breathing helps in the removal of toxins and waste products from the body. It also serves to provide more oxygen and nutrient material for both the mother and child. On another level, deep breathing helps the concentration of the mind, purifies and calms the nervous system, and improves the chemical environment within the body of the pregnant woman. Since pranayama relaxes both the body and mind, it can help to decrease labor pains, which take over the mind at the time of delivery. In addition to helping the delivering mother to bear the pain, deep breathing aids in pushing the child out of the womb. Because of its rhythmic nature, pranayama sets up a rhythm in the system that helps harmonize the bodily forces. The combination of a healthy spine—made strong by massage—and rhythmic breathing takes away the fear that produces tension and blocks the natural process of labor. Pain is a natural device created by nature to aid the birth and cannot be completely eliminated, but massage and pranayama allow the pregnant woman to tolerate the pain and maintain a state of emotional balance.

After the first three months of pregnancy, massage of the pregnant woman should incorporate relaxation exercises. Many women experience intensified emotions during pregnancy, especially after the third month; they also can become subject to sudden depression. Relaxation helps to minimize this emotional stress. After completing each segment of the back massage—the pelvis, the spine, and the back—the practitioner should give the recipient a certain amount of time to practice simple deep-breathing exercises as described above or one of the following relaxation exercises: *yoga nidra* (yogic sleep), shavasana (the corpse posture), counting of the breaths, or mantra repetition.

Yoga nidra is a practice that brings on a state of deep relaxation. To achieve this state, an awareness of the body induces relaxation of the mind. This is done by autosuggestion: the mind is engaged in observing the body as it progressively relaxes, from the toes to the top of the cranium. To practice the yogic posture shavasana, the recipient simply lies on her back, legs and arms slightly separated from the body, and breathes slowly using the full abdominal breath. (See page 51 for a transcription of directions for shavasana.) Another easy relaxation technique is simply to count one's breaths. Ideally this is done in a 1:4:2

ratio. For example, inhale to the count of two; hold to the count of eight; exhale to the count of four. Alternately, combining the repetition of a mantra with the breath can be very helpful in inducing deep relaxation. Even simple awareness of deep breathing will help calm the mind and nervous system and avert an emotional crisis.

The alternation of the three phases of back massage with the relaxation methods just described is quite beneficial. It will help with the release of growth hormones in the correct proportion and will help in the proper development of the fetus. This dynamic combination provides vitality to the expectant mother, making her able to provide pranic force and oxygen to the developing fetus more efficiently. It also increases the peace and harmony in both the mother and child.

STAGES OF PREGNANCY

First and Second Month

According to the *Sushruta Samhita,* during the first month of pregnancy only a gelatinous substance is formed in the womb. This information, as well as much of the other information provided by Sushruta in this text, is corroborated by medical science. Sushruta states that approximately six or seven days after conception, the new organism embeds itself in the lining of the uterus. In about the seventh week the embryo assumes a recognizable form. He goes on to say that in the second month the embryo takes a shape that is either lumplike, in the case of a male child, or elongated, which indicates a female child. According to medical science, the limbs appear as tiny buds on the embryo when it is less than a month old, and the heart starts beating a few days before the end of the first month.

In sum, it is during the seventh week—the end of the second month of pregnancy—that the human embryo assumes a recognizable form. By this time the brain has already been formed, with the capability of coordinating the other organs of the body through electrical impulses. Growth during this period is rapid but irregular. The skeleton begins to develop after the forty-sixth to forty-eighth day, which means that the body of the pregnant woman needs more calcium and other minerals.

During this time proper massage of the back and abdominal region is necessary, and the expectant mother should relax and only engage in light housework. She should also practice deep-breathing exercises and meditation whenever possible.

The massage practitioner should spend more time massaging the back, as well as the thighs, calves, ankles, and feet. The use of oil should be minimized since oil needs more rubbing to be absorbed into the body, causing possible strain to a pregnant woman's body and disrupting her normal breathing pattern. Instead of applying oil directly onto the body, the practitioner's hands should be lubricated with just enough oil to allow smooth rubbing, pressing, kneading, and squeezing of the body. In India, mustard oil is commonly used both before and after delivery, although peanut oil and coconut oil are also used. The practitioner should follow the mother's preferences if another oil is preferred for fragrance or other reasons.

Third and Fourth Months

During the third month the fetus develops muscles and can move its limbs. The movement is feeble, however, and the mother cannot feel it.

In the fourth month, according to the *Sushruta Samhita,* all the limbs and organs of the embryo become stronger and the fetus is endowed with consciousness, owing to the formation of the viscous of the heart. The heart is the seat of consciousness; by this vehicle the fetus expresses its desire for sensory pleasures—such as things of taste and smell—through the longing of its mother. This month is important for the practitioner because from now on he or she has to obey the instructions of the expectant mother about oil selection and fragrance, since the child's preferences may be known through the mother's.

Soothing and relaxing massages should be given during this time to the waist, back, spine, and abdominal regions. The legs and shoulders also need some rubbing, pressing, and kneading. By the end of the fourth month the fetus gains about half the height it will be at birth.

Fifth and Sixth Months

By the fifth month, movements of the fetus can be clearly felt and detected by the expectant mother. During the sixth month the child is endowed with mind; it sleeps, wakes up aware of its subconscious existence, and changes positions. It also begins to accumulate fat and develop fingernails. The activity inside the womb increases during this period; the child grows to about a foot long and weighs between twelve and twenty ounces.

In the sixth month, the faculty of cognition is developed. The child is able to respond to the external environment of the womb. Massage of the waist, back, and spine should be done gently and for a longer period of time, and the massage should conclude with the rubbing and pressing of shoulders and calves. The abdominal region should not be massaged after the fourth month; it should only be rubbed very gently.

Seventh, Eighth, and Ninth Months

During the seventh month, all the limbs are clearly developed. The last three months are the time of completion of the physical aspect of development in the uterus—the child grows, gains weight, and acquires muscular control. The purpose of massage and breathing exercise during this time period is to remove tension and stress, strengthen the spine, and remove toxins.

Massage enhances circulation and helps to purify the blood. Deep-breathing exercises and pranayama, combined with massage, provide vitality as well as the oxygen and antibodies required for the immune system of the child. Massage should continue up to the beginning of the labor pains. During labor the expectant mother should be given massage for relaxation to reduce fear and the tensions and blockages produced by fear. The laboring woman may be massaged on the shoulders and neck to reduce the tension felt in giving birth. This area should be treated more gently than before labor pains began. On the other hand, her back, waist, and pelvis can be massaged more deeply than was advised after the fourth month and before the onset of labor. The legs and calves should not be massaged during labor.

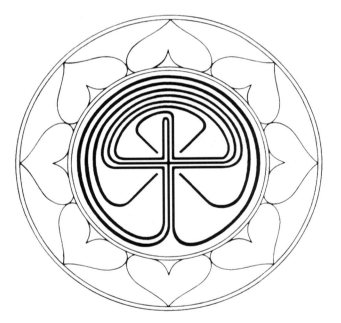

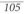
105

The expectant mother should feel safe and protected at this time. She should be asked to visualize the child's birth or to concentrate on a yantra for the childbirth. Either of these forms of concentration helps promote a quick delivery, if done once the real labor pains start. The yantra in figure 105 is often drawn with a red paste onto a metal plate and set in front of the laboring woman. Meditation on this form helps the woman overcome her fears by diverting her attention from her pain. The resulting relaxation allows the child to be born more easily.

After Delivery

Following delivery of the child, the new mother should be allowed to relax for three or four days. After this time, massage and deep-breathing exercises should be resumed and continued for forty days. While this time period can be prolonged, it should not be reduced. In India, both the newborn and the mother are given massage as regularly as they are given food and nourishment. The value of massage as a cleansing tool is especially important at this time, since neither the mother nor child can engage in any strenuous physical exercise.

A woman's body undergoes a lot of physical and mental strain during the process of delivery. There is pain before and after delivery. In addition to massage of the abdomen, postdelivery massage that focuses on the calves, waist, back, neck, and shoulders helps the new mother's body to reorganize itself and to relax, thus promoting a quick recovery. During the last four months of pregnancy, the musculature of the abdominal region gets stretched as the fetus continues to grow. Regular massage with oil can help the muscles regain their natural shape after delivery.

In modern times, new mothers find they cannot afford forty days of rest; such rest is only possible for mothers living in extended families. When this rest is denied, problems related to stress and strain are created, which in turn destroy a woman's natural romantic feelings. While the social structure women live in may have changed with the changing economy, the postdelivery abdominal musculature of women has not changed. Today we may have better standards of living, but we are losing our sound mental and physical health. However the task of recovery is accomplished, we cannot deny a new mother the rest she so dearly needs. In the Hindu tradition, the new mother is considered to be in a process of natural cleansing for the forty days following delivery. She is not allowed to worship or to cook during this period. After the cleansing period has ended, she is given a bath. This serves as an official declaration that she is fit to resume her household work and her normal routines of worship. During her forty-day rest period, she is given nourishing food, light exercises to practice, and massage. In this day and age, we need to take care not to destroy our marital life by denying the new mother her most desired rest and her oil massage. These will help speed her recovery and lift her spirits.

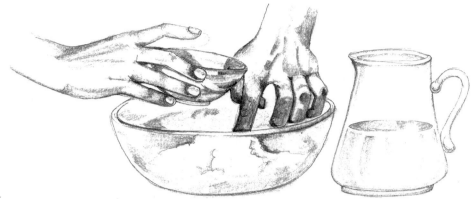

106

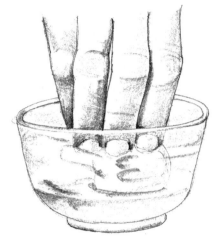

107

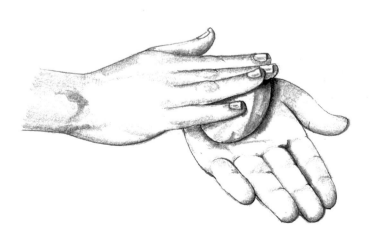

108

Chapter Eight

Massage of Infants

The massage of newborn babies has a long tradition in India. Like massage of the new mother, massage of the newborn—initially, at least—is also a necessary phenomenon. According to the *Sushruta Samhita,* a cleansing massage is recommended just after birth—before the umbilical cord is cut—to clean the shreds of the membrane covering the infant's body. Traditionally this is done by rolling a dough ball over the body. A soft dough ball, about the size of a lemon, is made from fresh, finely ground whole wheat flour and water. As the ball is being formed, a little almond oil is added to make it smooth and nourishing for the baby's skin (figs. 106, 107, and 108). (This oil supplements the oil already present in the wheat grain itself.) A dash of turmeric may also be added to the flour to help strengthen the skin and protect it from infection. Instead of rubbing the body of the newborn baby with one's hands, it is gently rubbed with this dough ball. (If these ingredients are not available, any clean, soft cloth may be used. Oil does not need to be applied to the cloth.) The texture of the dough ball, which gets warmed by contact with human hands, is very similar in temperature and texture to the mother's flesh. Just before rubbing the ball on the infant's body it is dipped in a bit of almond oil, which causes the membrane shreds to stick to the dough ball. After this process is complete, the mouth of the infant is cleansed of mucus. The *Sushruta Samhita* recommends using ghee (clarified butter will do) and rock salt. The cleaning of the mouth is done by lubricating the fingers with ghee that has been combined with a pinch of rock salt, then carefully inserting the lubricated fingers in the mouth and cleansing the mucus from the mouth. The *Sushruta Samhita* continues to say that after this mouth cleaning, a linen pad soaked in clarified butter should be applied to

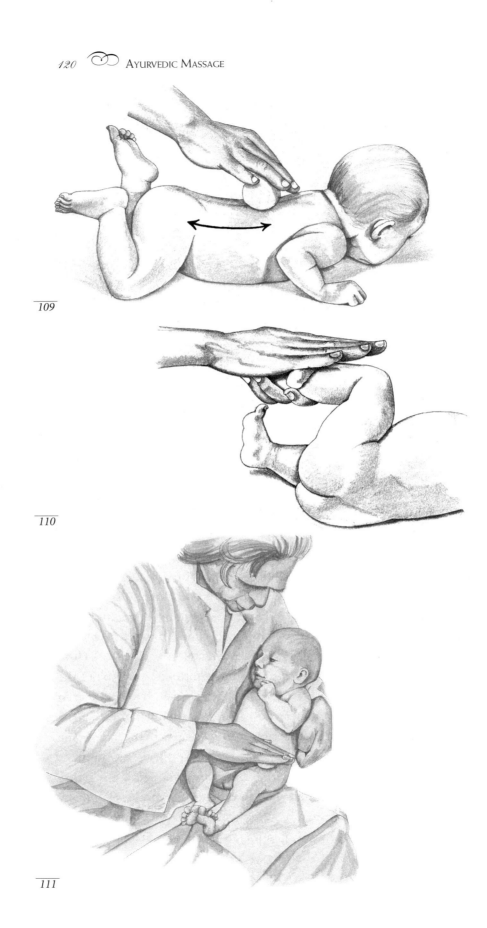

109

110

111

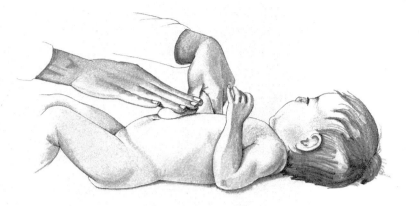

the head of the newborn baby. Then the umbilical cord, after having been pulled gently so that it is drawn slightly away from the abdomen, should be ligatured with one end of a string at a point eight fingerwidths from the navel, and the other end of the string tied around the infant's neck. Up to this point the umbilical cord is essential to the existence of the child, as all important nadis are connected with it. If the cord is cut without having a support on the side where it is connected to the navel, it will fall down. But when the other end of the string is tied around the neck of the baby, the thread supports that part of the cord and it does not need to be touched with fingers or tongs. Then the umbilical cord should be severed immediately above the ligature.

For the first six days after birth, the infant is cleaned with a freshly made dough ball before its bath. Rubbing with the dough ball enhances circulation, helps in the expulsion of toxins, and aids the digestive system of the baby. Usually the practitioner who is massaging the new mother massages the infant as well.

On the seventh day after birth, actual massage with the dough ball begins and continues for three weeks. Before this time the dough ball is used as an applicator for oil to cleanse the infant's body. Massage with the dough ball differs from cleansing because in the massage the infant is repeatedly rubbed in the same areas with the dough ball, and moderate pressure is used (figs. 109, 110, 111, and 112). Once the infant's skin becomes a bit red and the body temperature rises, the bath may be given. The dough ball should be dipped in oil every now and then. The absorption of the oil into the infant's skin helps to keep the three doshas in proper balance.

Massage with the hands begins when the infant is one month old, after sufficient oil has been absorbed and the baby's body has become strong. Massage oils, such as mustard, sesame, or coconut, are usually used in India. Mustard oil is used in winter, coconut oil in summer, and sesame in spring and fall. Mustard oil, however, can be irritating to the delicate skin of some babies, and for them only almond, coconut, or sesame oils are recommended.

The dough ball is now used only as a cleansing tool, and only as needed. It can be helpful in removing hairs from the infant's body. If the dough ball massage is not done during the first three months, unnecessary hairs can sometimes grow on the face, arms, legs, and back; this can bring embarrassment to the child, especially the girls, in adolescence.

Massage done with the hands, using the oil appropriate to the season and the dosha, is continued every day for three months. During the three-month period, the practitioner should manipulate the infant's arms and legs to engage and exercise the muscles. Also during this time, the practitioner should spend more time massaging the spine, back, neck, and waist regions and the hands and feet, because these parts need to gain strength to support the body. Once the baby starts lifting its head on its own and supporting its body weight on its arms, these practices may be discontinued. The massage of the spine, however, still remains an important aspect of the baby's massage. The genitals and anus of the infant should be massaged daily with oil to help prevent infections. With a male infant, the foreskin of the penis should be pulled back and oil should be applied on the exposed area to help prevent fungal infection.

A cotton or linen pad soaked in oil (discussed on page 88) should be applied to the head for the first four to six weeks only. After that time, the infant's movements make it too difficult to keep the pad in place. This practice is very beneficial because it removes dryness of the scalp and strengthens the hair roots. After the six-week period, oil is still applied to the head region during massage.

During the first three months, the infant should be handled carefully and any discomfort should be avoided. Massage should not be done in the open air, unless there is enough sun and warmth. The baby should not be scolded or suddenly roused from sleep lest it becomes frightened. The baby should also not be picked up or put down suddenly; this could lead to a derangement of vayu (air) in the body. Any attempt to seat a child before it has become strong enough to support itself may lead to a hunchback condition (kyphosis).

According to the *Sushruta Samhita*, a child should not be left alone in an unclean or unholy place; it should not be left under the sky (in an uncovered place), or over undulating ground; it should not be exposed to heat, storms, rain, dust, smoke, or cold water. A child that is raised in keeping with these principles, and with love and affection, becomes healthy, cheerful, and intelligent.

Daily massage of a baby should be continued for eighteen months. After this time, massage can be given on alternate days. If it is possible to continue with a daily massage routine, however, it will aid in making the child strong and happy.

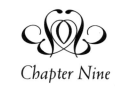

Chapter Nine

Beauty Massage

From the dawn of civilization man has been searching for a miraculous ambrosia that would prevent decay, and even death, of the body. Sages and seers prescribed simple *yamas* (rules of conduct) and *niyamas* (rules of inner control) to maintain a balanced body chemistry. Yoga postures and pranayama (breathing exercises) were used to maintain virility, vitality, flexibility of the spine, and health of the bones, musculature, ligaments, and nerves. Meditation and other means of achieving deep relaxation, such as massage, were also recommended to increase one's health and radiance. The *Sushruta Samhita* states that for those seeking perfect health and a sound body, *abhang* or anointing of the body is prescribed. Vagbhata mentions in his *Ashtanga Hridaya* that massage is called *ayu-kar,* meaning that which increases longevity. According to Vagbhata, when all these practices were combined they could help a man live a happy, healthy, inspired, and long life.

Qualities such as fear, passion, anger, greed, malice, jealousy, envy, selfishness, and sloth constantly spoil body chemistry. When the body gets overloaded with toxins, these negative qualities begin to influence the cells of the body, and in turn the natural shape and texture of the skin is destroyed. The spine becomes tense and the body's natural radiance is lost; the body becomes rough looking and ugly.

The spine is the center of the nervous system and all neuromotor actions. Its shape plays an important role in the shape of the body. If the spine is not in good configuration, the body will suffer. The spine is connected with all internal organs and is the seat of the primary psychic centers. If the spine is massaged properly, growth hormones are released, which play a key role in physical beauty. Before age forty-five, everything needed for a person's well-being is contained inside and massage simply enhances the circulation of those nutrient materials from within. However, after the age of forty-five, minerals and vitamins need to be added to one's regular diet in the form of gem oxides, gem powders, and rasayanas, which are rejuvenating tonics made from medicinal herbs and plants. Massage of the spine can cure many problems caused by deranged vata and kapha.

By practicing nonviolence, contentment, tolerance, and forgiveness and abstaining from malice, jealousy, and envy; by maintaining a good vegetarian diet; and by employing massage, breathing exercises, and meditation, one can help the body restore, to a certain extent, its natural radiance and beauty. The practice of massage alone, without implementing a change in habits and lifestyle, is not sufficient. If the degeneration of the body is due to aging, then special nourishing and rejuvenating preparations made from medicinal herbs, gems, and powders must be used in a beauty massage. If the premature aging and decay is caused by disease, then the therapeutic cure for the condition must be followed before implementing the beauty massage.

Beauty massage can help those who have their health and live in accordance with the yamas and niyamas as just mentioned. It can also help those recovering from illness, those whose skin has become rough due to vata derangement, and those who have aged prematurely because of the stress and strain of life. Beauty massage can produce miracles for young, energetic people. The massage described in this section is actually for people of all ages, providing they eat the proper foods, take adequate rest, and practice deep-breathing exercises.

Elderly persons who abstain from intoxicants and incorrect foods and who exercise will look younger than their age not only during the course of treatment but long afterward, providing they maintain these good habits.

Dietary Preparation

The beauty massage treatment is a forty-day course. At least two weeks before beginning the treatment, meat, chicken, fish, and eggs should be renounced. The first day of the treatment routine starts with the taking of a purgative. For the next three or four days, eat only soups and *khichari*, preferably an equal mixture of moong dal and rice.[*] For the rest of the treatment routine follow a vegetarian diet, eating plenty of fruits, vegetables, nuts, seeds, milk, cheese, and cream. (Those with weight problems, however, should use dairy foods in sparing amounts.) Herbal teas are useful to help elimination and purify the blood

---

[*] Khichari is a rice and dal dish. For a khichari recipe, see *The Healing Cuisine* by Harish Johari (Rochester, Vermont: Healing Arts Press, 1994).

chemistry. By following this dietary regime, the effects of the beauty massage will manifest more quickly.

At one time a popular practice among kings and queens in India was the taking of a bath with raw milk and rubbing the body with malai (the skin from boiled milk), cream, or unprocessed butter.* People born during an ascending cycle of the moon should try it two weeks before this cycle, starting the morning following the darkest night. The reverse applies to those born during a descending cycle.

While the diet and facials described here can be self-administered and will yield improved skin texture and tone, the full benefits of a beauty massage cannot be realized without a spine, neck, and shoulder massage from a qualified practitioner.

ENVIRONMENT FOR BEAUTY-MASSAGE TREATMENT

The practitioner should be a tender and happy person. The treatment should be given in a warm, enclosed, and cozy space. A good environment, made even more pleasing by the presence of flowers and the use of incense, should be created. It should be well protected from interruptions in the form of telephone calls or frequent visitors. Joyful and relaxing music should be played during the massage.

The practitioner should not talk too much, but should be informed enough about the oils and pastes to explain their benefits if the recipient asks. All mask preparations should be made fresh the night before by the practitioner and stored in glass jars in a cool, dry place to avoid fermentation. Each day the beauty massage should begin with the recipient having the right nostril open and dominant. If this is not the case, the recipient needs to lie on his or her left side, in the fetal posture, until the right nostril opens.† (See the discussion of the relationship between the nostrils and brain-hemisphere dominance on page 52.)

The beauty massage takes at least 80 minutes, and up to 120 minutes for those treatments that require special application and rubbing-off procedures. (Those special treatments are described on pages 126 through 135.) Woven into the beauty massage are small relaxation periods which take a total of 35 to 40 minutes. Altogether the practitioner should allow 2 to 2½ hours for the beauty massage treatment, not counting the bath or shower that follows. While the time for relaxation could be reduced, the results would not be the same.

---

* The malai, cream, and unprocessed butter was rubbed on the face, neck, hands, breasts, and feet; if butter was used, it was rubbed on the whole body.

† When the right nostril is open, the body can absorb the nourishing ingredients of the masks and oils more easily. Having this nostril open also protects the body against cold and aggravation of kapha.

The forty-day beauty treatment routine is outlined in the table below. The procedures and formulas are described in the pages that follow.

Forty-Day Beauty Treatment Routine

Day	Procedure	Formula	Procedure Time (min.)	Relaxation Time (min.)
1	Beauty massage	Basic oil formula	80	40
2	Full-body ubtan and body rub	Ubtan formula # 5 and relaxation followed by basic oil formula	100	40
3	Beauty massage	Basic oil formula	80	40
4	Clay bath and beauty massage	Wet clay and relaxation followed by basic oil formula	120	40
5	Beauty massage and facial ubtan	Basic oil formula followed by ubtan formula # 2	90	40
6	Beauty massage and facial mask	Basic oil formula followed by almond and cream mask	100	40
7	Beauty massage and facial mask	Basic oil formula followed by almond and cream mask	90	40
8	Beauty massage	Basic oil formula	80	40
9	Full-body ubtan	Ubtan formula # 5 followed by relaxation and body rub with oil	100	60
10	Beauty massage	Basic oil formula	80	40
11–21	Beauty massage	Raw milk body formula	80	40
22	Full-body ubtan and body rub	Ubtan formula # 5 and relaxation followed by raw milk body formula	100	60
23	Beauty massage and facial mask	Raw milk body formula followed by almond and cream mask	90	40
24	Beauty massage	Raw milk body formula	80	40
25	Beauty massage and facial mask	Raw milk body formula followed by almond and cream mask	90	40
26–28	Beauty massage	Raw milk body formula	80	40
29	Beauty massage and facial mask	Raw milk body formula followed by almond and cream mask	90	40

30	Full-body ubtan and body rub	Ubtan formula #5 followed by relaxation and raw milk body formula	100	60
31	Beauty massage	Raw milk body formula	80	40
32–34	Beauty massage	Basic oil formula	80	40
35–40	Full body ubtan and body rub	Ubtan formula #5 followed by relaxation and basic oil formula	100	60

THE BEAUTY MASSAGE SEQUENCE

For a description of the massage techniques, such as tapping, kneading, rubbing, and squeezing, see pages 47–48.

Spine (15 minutes' massage; 10 minutes' rest)

After checking that the recipient's right nostril is dominant (see page 52), have him or her lie face down on the massage table. Oil your hands and begin by tapping the base of the spine gently with your palms. Then knead the area with your fingertips and rub along the spine with the thumbs and wrists of both hands, always moving toward the head. Continue for 15 minutes. Cover the recipient with a sheet or towel made of linen or cotton, and rest together in shavasana (see page 51) for 10 minutes. During this time you may talk about such things as right living habits, health, or the effect foods have on beauty and radiance. You may also simply relax together.

Arms and Hands (30 minutes' massage; 10 minutes' rest)

Oil your palms again and begin the tapping, kneading, and rubbing process. Start at the shoulder blades and work down to the fingers. Spend more time on the joints—shoulder, elbow, wrist, finger—than on the musculature in between. When you have done one entire arm, flex the elbow and rotate the shoulder joint; make a crisscross movement down the whole arm to the fingers. Finish by massaging each finger independently and then gently rubbing a drop of oil onto each nail. When both arms have been done, cover the recipient with a linen sheet or towel again, and rest for 10 minutes.

Shoulders and Neck (5 minutes' massage; 5 minutes' rest)

Applying a little more than bearable pressure, press from the shoulder joint to the neck a few times. Then press on the neck muscles, working from the base of the neck to the occiput. Repeat these steps, rubbing oil into the muscles until it is absorbed. Do not work on shoulders and neck longer than 5 minutes. This segment can be followed by a 5-minute optional relaxation period.

Face (30 minutes' massage; 10 minutes' rest)

Ask the recipient to turn over onto his or her back. Choose one of the following facial formulas: a small amount of the basic oil formula, the raw milk facial formula, or the cream from raw milk. Use only one of these and use it each time throughout the forty-day course of treatment. Following the face massage, the practitioner may apply a mask. Once it begins to dry, the mask should be removed and the beeswax cream can be applied.

Begin by rubbing the facial formula of choice onto the lower jaw and chin for about 3 minutes, to allow nutrients to be absorbed by the skin. Gentle pressure with the palms on the lower jaw and chin is helpful for relieving tension. Then rub both cheeks in gradually expanding concentric circles, to enhance circulation and help remove wrinkles. The cheeks can be gently pinched, pressed, and pulled a few times with the fingertips. Ask the recipient to take a deep breath and hold the air inside, so the cheeks softly expand. The cheek massage can continue as far as the temporomandibular joint area, in front of the ear. All parts of the face where wrinkles develop should be lifted by the fingers and rubbed. Wrinkles tend to form near the nose and around the eyes, forehead, and lips. *Husne yusuf* grass is a fantastic remedy for removing wrinkles. It can be made into a simple paste using a mortar and pestle and a little milk and applied directly, or used as part of a formula (see almond and cream mask, page 133).

Moving from the cheeks and jawbone, lightly rub the nose, then gently press across the closed eyelids and eye sockets. Palming the eyes for a few minutes can help induce deep relaxation. Then hold both eyebrows between the thumb and forefinger of each hand and press gently for their full length.

Since the forehead records our unfavorable thoughts and emotions, it often reveals wrinkles. The practitioner should lift the forehead skin lightly, and then massage around the forehead in small circles.

The face massage culminates with a heavy cream massage of the lips by the practitioner. Circular movements of the fingertip (clockwise with right hand, counterclockwise with left hand) are ideal. These small circles can also be applied to the cheeks, nose, and forehead. Just before covering the recipient with the sheet or towel, place a drop of pure rosewater, which has been stored in a cool place in a blue bottle, in each eye. Be certain that the rosewater is pure—that is, water distilled from rose petals, not the commonly found distilled water with a few drops of rose essence added. The latter is not good for the eyes.

HELPFUL TIPS

The following practices will supplement the effect of the beauty treatment and should be continued after the forty-day session is completed. In the evening before retiring the feet should be massaged, at least 10 minutes for each foot. Malai, the skin of boiled milk, should be gently rubbed into the face for 10 minutes before going to sleep. In the morning the malai is simply rinsed off with lukewarm water. The eyes then should be washed with fresh spring or well water, to which a few drops of rosewater have been added. This not only improves one's sight but lends a freshness to the eyes. Rosewater and cool water are cooling, and the eyes need cooling to become strong. In nature cures, the eyes are strengthened by the application of cold, wet cloth pads. After the eyes are treated, beeswax cream (see page 134) can be applied to the face.

Only creams made from herbs and pure oils and beeswax should be used on the face; synthetic cosmetics, moisturizers, and sprays should be abandoned. Generally the face should be washed with water that is cooler than the body temperature. When bathing, one should avoid applying warm water to the head, face, and eyes.

SPECIAL TREATMENTS

Clay Baths

In the clay-bath treatment, the body is covered from head to toe with a paste of wet clay. Just before it is completely dry, the clay is rubbed off with the practitioner's fingertips. Then the body is gently rubbed. When no trace of clay remains, the recipient assumes the shavasana pose for 40 minutes (see page 51). This is followed by a full-body rub with oil and a warm shower.

Ubtan

Ubtan is a paste made from nuts or flour to which other ingredients, such as oil and spices, are added. In India, ubtan is used as a part of the ceremonial massage given before a marriage. The bride and groom are each given an ubtan massage in their respective homes before the ceremony. This not only helps them relax but also gives them a healthy glow.

Soaps available on the market generally strip away the oils and natural chemicals on the skin. Soaps also desiccate the pores. Because ubtan is made from natural, nourishing ingredients, it provides a wonderful way to clean the skin and should be used instead of soaps. The turmeric in the ubtan formulas provides iodine in a form that can be absorbed directly through the skin. The flour and oil in ubtan serve to both cleanse and lubricate. Chickpea flour is especially beneficial for the skin; oils, in general, lend a smooth, healthy glow to the skin.

Initially the paste draws excess heat out of the body or face. After the paste begins to dry, the rubbing motion used to remove it restores the normal body temperature, enhances circulation, and draws fresh energy to the surface of the skin.

Utban can be applied to the face, upper body, or the entire body.

After removing the paste in a facial ubtan, splash the face with cool water to which a few drops of rosewater have been added. Then rinse with warm water (which may contain a few drops of freshly squeezed lemon juice, if desired). After patting dry, gently apply beeswax cream to the face.

In a body ubtan, a bath with cool or lukewarm water should be taken one hour after removing the paste from the body. Fresh lemon juice can be added to the bathwater. For the hour between the ubtan and the bath, a sunbath may be taken during winter. The face, however, should be shielded from direct sun. In the privacy of an indoor garden area the sun may be enjoyed during the relaxation periods for no more than 20 minutes.

The recipes for the ubtan formulas follow. For formula #1 through #5, mix ingredients into a thick paste, adding as much water as necessary. For formula #6 and #7, follow the instructions given.

UBTAN FORMULA #1: *FOR WHOLE-BODY UBTAN MASSAGE*

This formula provides enough for a whole-body ubtan.

> $1\frac{1}{2}$ teaspoons mustard oil
> 4 tablespoons chickpea flour
> 1 teaspoon turmeric powder

UBTAN FORMULA #2: *FOR GLOWING, SMOOTH SKIN*

This formula provides enough paste to cover the entire body.

> $1\frac{1}{2}$ teaspoons mustard or almond oil
> 4 tablespoons chickpea flour
> 1 teaspoon turmeric powder
> 1 tablespoon fenugreek powder

UBTAN FORMULA #3: *FOR RHEUMATISM*

Apply to painful places.

> $1\frac{1}{2}$ teaspoons olive oil
> $1\frac{1}{2}$ teaspoons fenugreek powder
> $\frac{3}{4}$ teaspoon mustard oil
> $\frac{1}{4}$ teaspoon garlic powder
> 4 tablespoons chickpea flour
> 1 teaspoon turmeric powder

UBTAN FORMULA #4: *FOR PIMPLES*

This formula provides enough for several facial applications. Apply directly to the pimple.

1½ teaspoons chiraunji (nut) paste
1½ teaspoons dried orange peel, powdered
1½ teaspoons coconut oil
1 tablespoon wheat germ oil
1 teaspoon turmeric powder
2 tablespoons chickpea flour
pinch of organic camphor powder

UBTAN FORMULA #5: *FOR FULL-BODY UBTAN*

This formula provides enough for the entire body.

4 tablespoons chickpea flour
2 tablespoons mustard or almond oil
1 teaspoon turmeric powder
1 teaspoon fenugreek powder
1 teaspoon wheat germ oil
¼ teaspoon rose oil

UBTAN FORMULA #6: *FOR FACIAL UBTAN*

This formula provides enough for one facial ubtan application.

1 tablespoon almond paste
1 tablespoon cashew paste
1½ teaspoons pistachio paste
1 tablespoon malai (skin of boiled milk)
1 tablespoon wheat germ oil
1 tablespoon rosewater
¼ cup red lentil paste (see lentil face mask, page 132)
chickpea flour (to thicken)

Soak almonds, cashews, and shelled pistachios separately in water to cover over-night. In the morning, drain each batch and remove the skin of the almonds. Using a mortar and pestle, make the amount of paste required for each nut.

Mix all the ingredients until they have the consistency of yogurt. To thicken, add a little chickpea flour.

This formula will keep in the refrigerator for 24 hours; after this time the flour and nut paste will turn sour. Make only enough for one treatment.

Ubtan Formula #7: *To make the skin glow*

The following method of making ubtan paste is mentioned in a scripture known as Vanaushadhi Chandrodaya. *This recipe makes enough for a full-body ubtan.*

> $^1/_4$ cup yellow or white mustard seeds
> 2 cups milk

Combine the mustard seeds and milk in a saucepan and bring to a boil. Lower the heat and simmer until the milk has evaporated completely. Place the boiled mustard seeds in the sun or on a room heater to dry. When thoroughly dry, render the seeds into a powder with a mortar and pestle, and store in a glass jar.

For an ubtan face mask, mix 3 level tablespoons of the sun-dried mustard seeds with a small amount of raw milk. Mix with a mortar and pestle until a paste the consistency of yogurt is formed.

This formula will keep in the refrigerator for 24 hours. After this time the raw milk will become sour.

Ubtan Formula #8: *To cleanse the face and reduce wrinkles*

> 1 lemon, juiced
> 1 tablespoon wheat germ oil
> $^1/_4$ cup whole wheat flour

Combine the lemon juice and wheat germ oil. Add flour until a paste the consistency of yogurt is formed. Use as a face mask. This formula will keep in the refrigerator for 36 hours. After this time the flour will ferment.

Formulas and Masks

Basic Oil Formula

> 2 cups sesame oil
> $^1/_2$ cup almond oil
> $^1/_2$ cup wheat germ oil
> $^1/_3$ cup sandalwood oil

Shake well and place in a clear glass bottle in the sun for 40 days. Store in a cool, dry place.

Lentil Facial Mask

> $^1/_2$ cup red lentils
> 2 cups of milk

Soak lentils overnight in milk. The following morning, grind the mixture into a paste, without adding water or milk. Apply the paste to the face. Before it dries completely, gently rub it off with your fingertips. Rinse the face with lukewarm water and rub it gently with a wet towel to enhance circulation.

RAW MILK FACIAL FORMULA

> $^1/_4$ cup of raw milk
> 1 teaspoon almond oil

Mix oil and milk well and massage into the face. Since it takes time for the oil to be absorbed, applications can be done in installments. The mixture can be stored in the refrigerator between installments.

RAW MILK BODY FORMULA

> 1 cup raw milk
> $^1/_2$ teaspoon almond oil
> $^1/_2$ teaspoon wheat germ oil

Combine and mix well.

ALMOND AND CREAM MASK

> 1 cup cow's cream (from raw milk is ideal)
> 1 cup yellow mustard seeds
> 7 almonds
> water (for soaking)
> 1 teaspoon husne yusuf grass[*]

Two days before the treatment, soak the mustard seeds in the cream overnight. If necessary, some raw milk can be added to the cream to increase the volume. The following morning, boil the mixture until the cream completely evaporates. Allow the seeds to dry in the sun. Set aside. (Enough mustard seeds are prepared to allow for several applications.)

One night before the treatment, soak the almonds in water overnight. In the morning, peel and render them into a paste with a mortar and pestle. Then pound 2 to 3 tablespoons of the sun-dried mustard seeds into a powder with a mortar and pestle; this should yield about 1 tablespoon of powder. (Place the remaining sun-dried seeds in a glass jar with a tight-fitting lid and store in a cool, dry, dark place.)

In a small bowl, combine the powdered mustard seed, powdered grass, and almond paste. Apply the paste to the face and, before it dries completely, gently rub it off with your fingertips. Rinse the face with lukewarm water and rub it gently with a wet towel to enhance circulation.

---

[*] Husne yusuf is a type of Persian grass that can be purchased from stores that carry Ayurvedic or Unani herbs.

Beeswax Cream

> 2 tablespoons sesame oil
> 2 tablespoons coconut oil
> 1 tablespoon mustard oil
> 4 tablespoons purified beeswax
> 1 tablespoon almond oil
> 1 tablespoon wheat germ oil
> $^3/_4$ tablespoon sandalwood oil
> $^3/_4$ tablespoon rose oil (optional)

Heat the sesame, coconut, and mustard oils in a saucepan. Liquefy the beeswax and add it to the oils. Remove from the heat and, when the mixture starts to cool, mix in the almond and wheat germ oil and stir. Add the sandalwood oil (and rose oil if desired, which soothes and nourishes the heart) and mix well. When the mixture is completely cool, store in a clear glass jar. This formula makes enough for one person to use daily for 6 months.

This cream should be used following any facial cleansing. It provides needed nutrients to the skin and is helpful in curing wounds, cuts, bites, burns, and even bed sores. It is equally effective on newborns and the very old. The beeswax protects the face from weather changes, pollution, and dust, yet does not clog the pores. In addition, it removes wrinkles, cures pimples and dry skin, and soothes rough skin.

Eye Remedies

Kajal is a popular eye remedy often made in the Indian countryside from the carbon deposit of the ghee lamp. To prepare it, people burn a cotton wick in a ghee lamp and place a clean silver (or bronze) plate or spoon across the flame. The carbon deposits are then gathered and mixed with a minute amount of ghee and a pinch of organic camphor.* The end result, a sticky paste the consistency of lipstick, is stored in tiny silver boxes. (Silver is ideal because it does not allow bacterial growth.) Kajal can also be made from burning a cotton wick in mustard oil. This procedure is common in India and the carbon collected from mustard oil is very medicinal.

To apply kajal, lightly touch the tip of the ring finger to the kajal. When a tiny amount adheres to the tip, apply it carefully to the full length of each eyelid. Kajal brightens the eyes, making them look more prominent and beautiful, but more importantly it has medicinal properties: it can cure many eye diseases, as well as improve sight and keep the eyes healthy. While a mild burning sensation

---

* A few drops of neem oil can be added to the ghee if desired.

and slight tearing may be experienced, this is caused by a chemical reaction that actually strengthens the eyes. Camphor is cooling and also excites the tear glands, helping the eyes to remain healthy.

Kajal should be applied to the eyes daily after washing the face in the morning. Men should apply kajal before retiring in the evening.

In India, men, women, and children of all ages, including newborns, wear kajal. Camphor, however, is not added to the formula for infants. Children wear kajal from the sixth day after birth until six years of age to protect the eyes. Manufactured kajal can be found in many Indian grocery stores in the West.

Surma is another eye remedy popular in India today. Surma is a powdered collyrium made by grinding antimony on a stone with herbs. Gem powders from pearl, emerald, and blue sapphire can also be used. Surma provides most of the same health benefits as kajal. Muslims apply it for religious reasons—the prophet Mohammad himself used surma. Surma is applied to the eyelids with a special silver or zinc rod.

Appendix

Marmas and Their Positions

adhipati: crown of the head

ani: above and lateral to the kneecap

ani: inside the arm, just above the elbow

ansa phalak: shoulder blades

ansa: shoulders

apalapa: above and to the side of the nipple area

apanga: outer corner of the eye

apastambha: between the nipple and the sternum

avarta: outer corner of the eyebrow

guda: tip of the tailbone

gulpha: ankle joint

hridayam: xiphoid process

indravasti: center of the calf

indravasti: middle of the forearm

janu: knee joint

kakshadhara: armpit

katika tarunam: base of the buttocks and the pelvic crest

krikatikas: base of the skull

kshipra: between the first and second toes

kshipra: between the thumb and first finger

kukundaraya: sacroiliac joints

kurchshira: heel of foot (posterior) and outer margin of foot (anterior)

kurchshira: middle of the wrist joint at the base of the thumb and just below the little finger

kurpara: inside the elbow joint

kuruchcha: above kshipra, root of the thumb

kuruchcha: ball of the foot

lohitaksha: inguinal region

lohitaksha: axial fold

manibandha: wrist joint

manya dhamni: side of the thyroid gland

nabhi: umbilicus

neel dhamni: front of the larynx

nitamba: outside angle of the iliac crest

parshva sandhi: above katika tarunam, at the high waist

phana: side of each nostril

shankh: the temple

simantakas: joints of skull bones

siramatrika: arteries on each side of neck

sringataka: on the soft palate

stanmula: below the nipple

stanrohita: above the nipple

sthapni: third eye

talhridaya: center of the sole of the foot

talhridayam: center of the palm

urvi: middle of the thigh

urvi: middle of the upper arm

utkshepa: above the ear

vastih: the bladder

vidhuram: below the ears

vitapam: root of the scrotum

vrihati: either side of the 10th thoracic vertebra

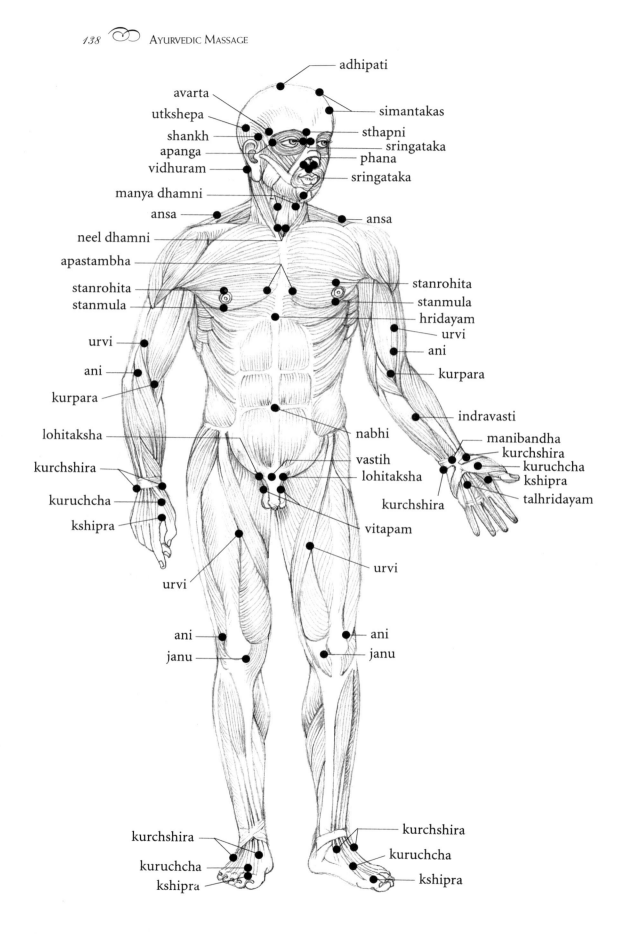

adhipati

avarta

utkshepa

shankh

apanga

vidhuram

manya dhamni

ansa

neel dhamni

apastambha

stanrohita

stanmula

urvi

ani

kurpara

lohitaksha

kurchshira

kuruchcha

kshipra

urvi

ani

janu

kurchshira

kuruchcha

kshipra

simantakas

sthapni

sringataka

phana

sringataka

ansa

stanrohita

stanmula

hridayam

urvi

ani

kurpara

indravasti

nabhi

manibandha

vastih

kurchshira

lohitaksha

kuruchcha

kshipra

kurchshira

talhridayam

vitapam

urvi

ani

janu

kurchshira

kuruchcha

kshipra

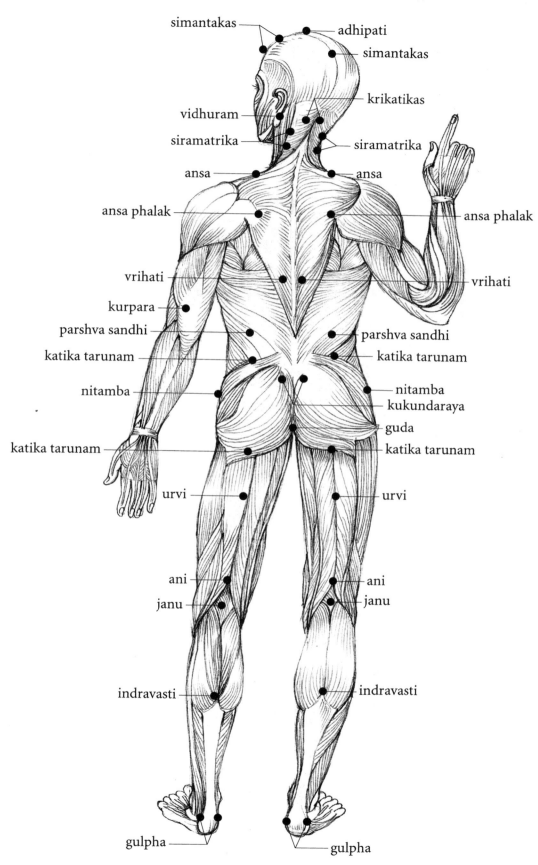

simantakas

adhipati

simantakas

krikatikas

vidhuram

siramatrika

siramatrika

ansa

ansa

ansa phalak

ansa phalak

vrihati

vrihati

kurpara

parshva sandhi

parshva sandhi

katika tarunam

katika tarunam

nitamba

nitamba

kukundaraya

guda

katika tarunam

katika tarunam

urvi

urvi

ani

ani

janu

janu

indravasti

indravasti

gulpha

gulpha

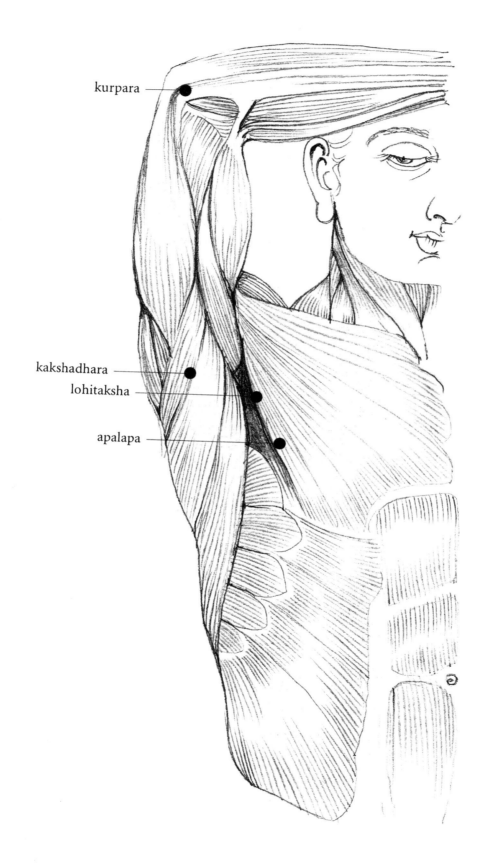

kurpara

kakshadhara

lohitaksha

apalapa

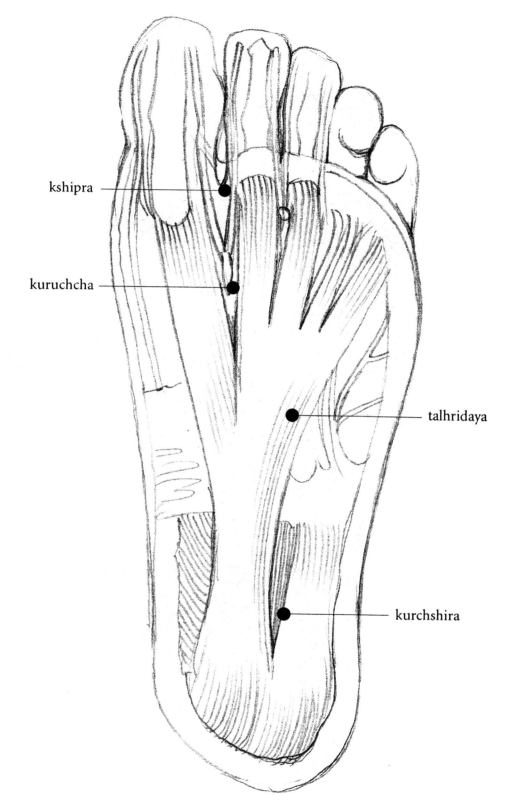

kshipra

kuruchcha

talhridaya

kurchshira

Glossary

In the definitions, words set in **bold face** are defined elsewhere in the Glossary.

Agni—The element of fire. One of the constituent elements (along with **apah** or water) of the **pitta** temperament.

Akash—The element of space. One of the constituent elements (along with **vayu** or air) of the **vata** temperament.

Apah—The element of water. One of the constituent elements (along with **agni** or fire) of the **pitta** temperament.

Asthi—Bones and teeth. Considered one of the seven main constituents, or **dhatus**, of the human body.

Ayurveda—*Ayu* (life), *veda* (knowledge). The ancient Indian science of "the knowledge of life" or "right living" for physical and mental well-being. The principles of Ayurveda are grounded in Vedic scriptures going back to 3000 B.C.

Brahmand—The fontanelle (the soft spot) at the top of the cranium, also known by yogis as the tenth gate. The brahmand absorbs pranic energy, solar radiation, and other forms of subtle energy present in the atmosphere. This spot, located eight fingerwidths above the third eye, is believed to be the seat of the Self. Anatomically, the brahmand is the hollow space between the two cerebral hemispheres. It is in the direct path of the **kundalini** energy that flows through the **sushumna**.

Chakras—Seven centers of activity of the vital life force (prana), specified on a physical level along the spinal column and interrelated with the nervous system and the endocrine glands. These subtle centers of consciousness are the link between the universal source of intelligence and the human body. Each chakra is associated with a particular state of consciousness. The chakras function in concert with one another; when this energy system is working well, the person experiences health and vitality of body and mind. Because of their correlations on a physical plane with the spine, the nervous system, and the endocrine glands, the chakras can be influenced by massage.

Dharma—Religious virtue.

Dhatus—The seven constituents of the human body, responsible for maintaining the functions of the organs, systems, and vital parts of the physical being. The seven dhatus are: **rasa** (fluids, hormones, lymph); **rakta** (blood); **mansa** (flesh, muscles, and cutis); **medha** (fat); **asthi** (bones and teeth); **majja** (marrow); and **shukra** (semen, vaginal fluids). The strength that comes from the dhatus gives the powers of tolerance, forbearance, and patience.

Doshas—The three body humors or temperaments. These are **vata** (wind), **pitta** (bile), and **kapha** (mucus). The doshas constitute the chemical nature of all living organisms. The three doshas produce various temperaments (**prakriti**) and physical types depending on their proportion in any one individual. Some people are clearly dominated by one of the three doshas while others are dominated by various combinations. Ayurveda advises eating foods and partaking of other activities that balance the intrinsic characteristics of the dominant dosha, rather than increasing or aggravating the existing condition. A harmonious balance of the three doshas is essential for the maintenance of physical and mental well-being.

Ghee—Sometimes referred to as clarified butter, ghee is made by churning yogurt into butter, which is then melted until the milk solids settle at the bottom of the pan. The butter is skimmed off the top and used for massage, cooking, and other applications.

Gunas—The three fundamental principles contained within all forms in the universe. These principles represent the natural evolutionary process through which the subtle becomes gross. These principles are **sattva** (essence, corresponding to **pitta**), **rajas** (activity, corresponding to **vata**), and **tamas** (inertia, corresponding to **kapha**). These are the three different phases through which all that exists passes. By keeping watch over one's actions and drives, one can, with the help of the knowledge of the gunas, assume responsibility for the development of one's own being. Keeping a watchful eye on one's habits—eating, sleeping, sexual—and on one's pattern of breathing, one discovers inner changes created by such things as food, colors, and sounds. One's own feelings are the clearest guide to the workings of the gunas within.

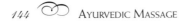

Hakim—A doctor of the Unani (Greek) system of medicine, which like Ayurveda utilizes the three humors, pressure points, herbs, spices, oils, and other natural techniques for wellness.

Hatha yoga—A yoga based on physical postures for uniting awareness of body and mind.

Kaddu oil—Oil extracted from the pumpkin seed.

Kapha—One of the primary **doshas** or temperaments formed by the elements of water and earth.

Kundalini—"Serpent power," spiritual energy that lies dormant at the base of the spine until it is awakened by yogic practices. The awakened kundalini energy ascends through the **sushumna** and passes through the first six chakras before it reaches its final abode, the seventh chakra at the **brahmand**. When this happens, the activities of the mind are completely suspended. One loses all sense of time and space, and identifications and false notions of the phenomenal world melt away.

Mahanarayana oil—A medicinal oil expressed from various plants.

Majja—Marrow. Considered one of the seven main constituents, or **dhatus**, of the human body.

Mansa—Flesh, muscles, and cutis. Considered one of the seven main constituents, or **dhatus**, of the human body.

Marmas—Pressure points in the Ayurvedic system of massage, occurring at the firm junctures of the five organic principles: **sira** (vessels), **mansa** (muscles), **snayu** (ligaments), **asthi** (bones), and **sandhi** (joints). These junctures form the seats of the vital life force or **prana**. At these junctures, the four classes of **sira** (vessels)—nerves, lymph, arteries, and veins—enter the organism to carry nutrients and moisture to the muscles, ligaments, bones, and joints.

Medha—Fat. Considered one of the seven main constituents, or **dhatus**, of the human body.

Meru danda—Spinal column.

Mudras—Hand postures traditionally used in sacred Indian dance.

Muqame makhsoos—Pressure points (Unani).

Nadi—A fine network of subtle nerves linked with the chakras. Pranic and psychic energy is absorbed and discharged through these subtle nerves.

Panchakarma—A special Ayurvedic massage technique for purification.

Pitta—One of the primary **doshas** or temperaments formed by the elements of fire and water.

Prakriti—The creative principle personified as Shakti, the Divine Mother. Prakriti also refers to an individual's temperament or **dosha**, which is determined at conception and unchangeable during one's lifetime. The prakriti is the basic chemical blueprint on which the organism has been constructed.

Prana—Vital life force. Ayurvedic massage increases the flow of prana in the body.

Prithvi—The element of earth. One of the constituent elements (along with **apah** or water) of the **kapha** temperament.

Purusha—The Father principle.

Rajas—One of the **gunas**, the three fundamental principles contained within all forms in the universe. Rajas, "activity," corresponds to **vata**.

Rakta—Blood. Considered one of the seven main constituents, or **dhatus**, of the human body.

Rasa—Fluids, hormones, and lymph. One of the seven main constituents, or **dhatus**, of the human body.

Sandhi—Joints.

Sattva—One of the **gunas**, the three fundamental principles contained within all forms in the universe. Sattva, "essence," corresponds to **pitta**.

Shukra—Semen and vaginal fluid. Considered one of the seven main constituents, or **dhatus**, of the human body.

Snayu—Ligaments.

Sneha—Oil.

Soma—The lunar principle of the organism.

Srotas—Channels in the body connected to the **marmas** and the internal organs, through which nutrient materials are supplied to the various tissues of the body. According to Ayurveda, the srotas are carriers of **vayu** (wind), **pitta** (bile), and **kapha** (mucus) and as such they sustain the human organism. Any obstruction in their flow can generate sickness. Through regular massage, the circulation of vital life fluids can be maintained.

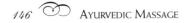

Sushumna—The main **nadi** or subtle channel known to yogis. According to tantric texts, prana travels through the sushumna from the pelvic plexus at the base of the spine to the hollow space between the two hemispheres of the brain. The sushumna passes through the **meru danda** (the spinal column); therefore, healthy alignment and functioning of the spine is crucial to optimal pranic flow in the body.

Swar yoga—A yoga based on the science of breath.

Tamas—One of the **gunas**, the three fundamental principles contained within all forms in the universe. Tamas, "inertia," corresponds to **kapha**.

Tejas—The fiery principle of the organism.

Til oil—Oil extracted from sesame seeds. Til oil is used frequently in Ayurvedic massage.

Tratak—Gazing at a candle flame until the eyes tear, a therapeutic practice in Ayurvedic medicine. Also a practice used to calm the mind in meditation.

Vaidya—An Ayurvedic doctor.

Vata—One of the three primary **doshas** or temperaments formed by the elements of ether and air.

Vayu—The element of air/wind. One of the constituent elements (along with **akash** or ether) of the **vata** temperament.

Vikriti—Imbalances to one's **prakriti** or individual temperament.

Sources of Supply

The following companies and individuals can provide supplies for Ayurvedic massage. Write or call for catalogs and mail order information.

The Ayurvedic Institute & Wellness
Center
P.O. Box 23445
Albuquerque, NM 87192-1445
(505) 291-9698
Herbs, oils, malas, including rudraksha
seeds

Bazaar of India Imports
1810 University Avenue
Berkeley, CA 94703
(800) 261-7662
Herbs, oils, gem powders and oxides

Dr. Abhai Kumar
Pocket B6
4263 Vasant Kunj
New Delhi 37, India
011-91-11-689-0810
Oil formulas, sun-treated oils

Maharishi Ayur-Ved
P.O. Box 49667
Colorado Springs, CO 80949-9667
(719) 260-5500
Oils, Ayurvedic skin and hair care
formulas, herbal nutrition formulas

Nature Care Products Company
6 Charles Park
Guilderland, NY 12084
(800) 923-9338
Ayruvedic massage oil, complete line of
Ayurvedic supplements, free brochure
with doshas test

Tej Ayurvedic Skin Care Clinic
162 W. 56th Street
New York, NY 10019
(212) 581-8136
Ayurvedic skin and hair care formulas

Index